The Path from Biomarker Discovery to Regulatory Qualification

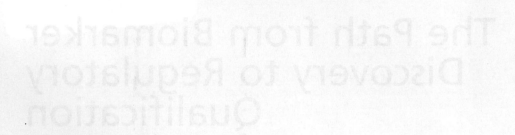

The Path from Biomarker Discovery to Regulatory Qualification

Federico Goodsaid

*Strategic Regulating Intelligence, Regulatory Affairs, Vertex
Pharmaceuticals, Washington DC, USA*

William B. Mattes

PharmPoint Consulting, Poolesville, Maryland, USA

ELSEVIER

Amsterdam • Boston • Heidelberg • London
New York • Oxford • Paris • San Diego
San Francisco • Singapore • Sydney • Tokyo

Academic Press is an imprint of Elsevier

Academic Press is an imprint of Elsevier
The Boulevard, Langford Lane, Kidlington, Oxford, OX5 1GB, UK
225 Wyman Street, Waltham, MA 02451, USA

Notice

No responsibility is assumed by the publisher for any injury and/or damage to persons or property as a matter of products liability, negligence or otherwise, or from any use or operation of any methods, products, instructions or ideas contained in the material herein. Because of rapid advances in the medical sciences, in particular, independent verification of diagnoses and drug dosages should be made

British Library Cataloguing-in-Publication Data
A catalogue record for this book is available from the British Library

Library of Congress Cataloging-in-Publication Data
A catalog record for this book is available from the Library of Congress

ISBN : 978-0-12-391496-5

For information on all Academic Press publications
visit our website at elsevierdirect.com

Typeset by TNQ Books and Journals
www.tnq.co.in

Printed and bound in the United States of America

13 14 15 16 17   10 9 8 7 6 5 4 3 2 1

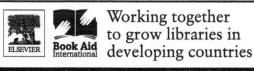

www.elsevier.com • www.bookaid.org

Contents

Section 3 Toxicogenomic Biomarkers

Section 4 Biomarkers of Drug Safety

Section 5 Consortia

Section 6 Path to Regulatory Qualification Process Development

Contributors

Shashi Amur
Office of Translational Sciences, Center for Drug Evaluation and Research, Food and Drug Administration, Silver Spring, Maryland, USA

Jiri Aubrecht
Pfizer Inc., Groton, Connecticut, USA

Joseph V. Bonventre
Renal Division, Department of Medicine, Brigham and Women's Hospital, Boston, Massachusetts, USA

Bruce D. Car
Pharmaceutical Candidate Optimization, Bristol-Myers Squibb, Inc., Princeton, New Jersey, USA

Jean-Philippe Couderc
University of Rochester Medical School, Rochester, New York, USA

Daniel C. Danila
Department of Medicine, Weill Cornell Medical College, New York, USA

Frank Dieterle
Novartis Pharma AG, Basel, Switzerland

Stephen T. Furlong
Astra Zeneca, Wilmington, Delaware, USA

Federico Goodsaid
Strategic Regulatory Intelligence, Regulatory Affairs, Vertex Pharmaceuticals, Washington DC, USA

Ernie Harpur
Institute of Cellular Medicine, Newcastle University, Newcastle, UK

Akihiro Ishiguro
PMDA Omics Project (POP), Pharmaceuticals and Medical Devices Agency (PMDA), Tokyo, Japan

Jeffrey Jacob
Cancer Prevention Pharmaceuticals and Critical Path Institute, Tuczon, Arizona, USA

Peter G. Lord
DiscoTox Ltd., Hebden Bridge, West Yorkshire, UK

William B. Mattes
PharmPoint Consulting, Poolesville, Maryland, USA

Raegan O'Lone
HESI, Washington DC, USA

Yasuto Otsubo
PMDA Omics Project (POP), Pharmaceuticals and Medical Devices Agency (PMDA), Tokyo, Japan

Syril Pettit
HESI, Washington DC, USA

Donald G. Robertson
Pharmaceutical Candidate Optimization, Bristol-Myers Squibb, Inc., Princeton, New Jersey, USA

Denise Robinson-Gravatt
Pfizer Inc., Groton, Connecticut, USA

Howard I. Scher
Memorial Sloan-Kettering Cancer Center, New York, USA

John R. Senior
Associate Director for Science, Food and Drug Administration (FDA), Silver Spring, Maryland, USA

Yoshiaki Uyama
PMDA Omics Project (POP), Pharmaceuticals and Medical Devices Agency (PMDA), Tokyo, Japan

Vishal S. Vaidya
Renal Division, Department of Medicine, Brigham and Women's Hospital, Boston, Massachusetts, USA; Harvard School of Public Health, Boston, Massachusetts, USA

Spiros Vamvakas
Head of Scientific Advice, European Medicines Agency, London, UK

Stephen A. Williams
Somatologic Inc., Boulder, Colorado, USA

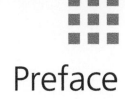

Preface

Successful work on drug development and regulatory review is often associated with strictly normative thinking. Drug development paths and regulatory policy can reach a level of acquiescence where the science which should drive these is only marginally integrated in them. The result of this process is drug development which yields less useful and less new drugs and regulatory review which mirrors and exacerbates the weaknesses of drug development.

The use of biomarkers in drug development at all levels is a powerful link to the science responsible for the identification, development and testing for transformative therapies. Whether in the assessment of drug safety or drug efficacy, in early or late development, in patient selection and characterization, and within a broad range of analytical platforms, biomarkers provide the information with which industry and regulators can determine whether a drug is safe and efficacious. While conventional definitions seek increasingly tenuous classifications for biomarkers, their shared value continues to be in what these biomarkers tell us about a drug and about what a drug can or cannot do in patients which should benefit from it. Results from biomarker measurements are not necessarily normative, and their inclusion in evolving concepts about why and when a drug is safe and efficacious continuously reminds us that we will only succeed with new therapies if we fully understand this information and the science behind it.

The collection of papers in this book includes contributions from scientists in academic institutions, pharmaceutical companies and regulatory agencies who have worked and continue to work on the best way to develop and use biomarkers from both the perspective of the critical path for drug development as well as from the perspective of the integration of these biomarkers in regulatory review. We hope that this snapshot of work carried out over the past decade will encourage further discussion about novel biomarkers and about how – and when – to make the best use of these powerful tools.

Federico Goodsaid and William B. Mattes

Introduction

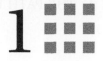

1

Biomarker Applications in the Pharmaceutical Industry

William B. Mattes

PHARMPOINT CONSULTING, POOLESVILLE, MARYLAND, USA

The 'explosion' of biomarker research is at least partially a semantic contrivance: as Ian Dews and others have noted; 'biomarkers' are not new [1]. Rather, as Dews notes, 'the word gave a long-overdue name' to characteristics noted and monitored by the health care profession for at least three millennia for the purposes of diagnosis or prognosis. Indeed, monitoring the pulse for the purpose of assessing the degree of injury is mentioned in the Edwin Smith Papyrus, describing Egyptian medical practice ca. 1500 BCE [2], and uroscopy as a 'science' is considered to date from Hippocrates [3]. The often quoted definition of the word, developed by the Biomarkers Definitions Working Group in 2001, is:

> *'a characteristic that is objectively measured and evaluated as an indicator of normal biological processes, pathogenic processes, or pharmacologic responses to a therapeutic intervention' [4].*

One might debate as to whether early uroscopy and the evaluation of pulse were 'objectively measured', yet certainly the definition applies to endpoints described prior to the first published use of the word 'biomarker'. That distinction goes to a 1977 paper examining the hypothesis that serum ribonuclease levels were a 'biomarker' of myeloma tumor cells [5]. However, the first publication in PubMed associated with biomarker as an index term dates to a 1947 study of fetuin-A [6], which more recently has been shown to serve as a 'biomarker' of coronary artery disease [7] and neurodegenerative disease [8]. Thus, while there has been an 'explosion' of publications using the term 'biomarker', it was preceded by an 'explosion' of publications examining endpoints indexed as biomarkers (Fig. 1.1), which even in 2009 surpassed by a factor of 10 the number of publications actually using the term. The point is that 'biomarkers' have only recently received <u>intentional</u> discussion of their discovery, definition, application, and qualification.

With the advent of technologies that allowed the precise determination of DNA sequence, and gene expression, a new form of biomarker entered the pantheon – the genomic, or pharmacogenomic, biomarker. While genetic disorders such as Down's syndrome could be characterized on a gross chromosomal level, determination of genetic polymorphisms, i.e., inter-individual variations in the sequence of genes, allowed for the

The Path from Biomarker Discovery to Regulatory Qualification. http://dx.doi.org/10.1016/B978-0-12-391496-5.00001-6

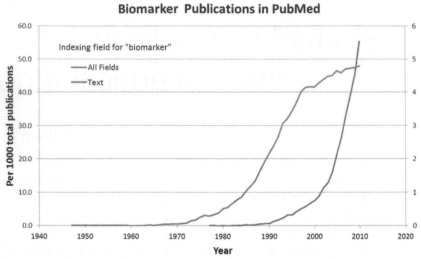

FIGURE 1.1 Biomarker publications indexed in PubMed. Numbers were determined using Alexandru Dan Corlan. Medline trend: automated yearly statistics of PubMed (http://dan.corlan.net/medline-trend.html).

correlation of DNA sequence variations with phenotypes relevant to disease and drug treatment. The problem of anticipating individual disease susceptibility or therapy response seemed to become tractable, as the tools gave clear, binary answers as to whether a given gene locus has a particular DNA sequence. In the 1990s the impact of genetic polymorphisms on drug metabolism in both animals and humans became clear and resulted in considerable research. Combined with the ancillary techniques for determining the individual enzymes responsible for a given drug's biotransformation in both preclinical species and in humans, pharmacogenomic approaches offered the promise of tailoring drug development programs such as to avoid or minimize the role of inter-individual variation in ADME (absorption, distribution, metabolism and excretion). The interest in the drug development community led to a survey of industry practices [9], an International Conference on Harmonization (ICH) guideline on definitions and sample handling [10], and guidance documents published by both the European Medicines Agency (EMA) [11] and the US Food and Drug Administration (FDA) [12]. The latter document suggests principles for the use of such pharmacogenomic biomarkers in early (i.e., exploratory) clinical studies, such as identifying populations that may require dosing adjustments or groups that might be at high risk for drug–drug interactions. The document also notes that such pharmacogenomic biomarkers may also include those other than for drug ADME, for example genetic variations in the drug target, and early clinical studies could identify those genetic variants most likely to respond to therapy, and use that information for patient enrichment strategies [13] in later clinical trials. The guidance acknowledges that in many cases samples may be collected during a given clinical trial and pharmacogenomic analysis conducted retrospectively to determine possible causes for toxicity or lack of efficacy. Indeed the industry predilection for retrospective, in contrast to prospective, analysis of pharmacogenomic biomarkers is echoed in an analysis of industry practices over the time frame 2003–2008 [14].

The relative caution applied to the application of pharmacogenomic biomarkers may reflect a more general caution in applying relatively novel biomarkers, particularly in regard to clinical trial design. Indeed such designs that can incorporate biomarker analysis as a variable in addition to the treatment variable have been the subject of many publications [15–18]. However, as noted above, 'biomarkers' have been discovered and applied for millennia, and their use qualified through a variety of approaches. While it is not the intent of this chapter to discuss qualification, it is the intent of this book to present examples of the approaches that have recently been used to do that.

The history of biomarkers reflects the inherent assumption that any given biomarker was almost certainly suitable for only a limited number of uses or applications. Such applications have been reviewed and classified in many publications and books, but for the purposes of this book it is worthwhile to consider the various types of biomarkers and applications, as these classifications have impact on the approaches taken toward qualifying a type of biomarker for a type of application.

Before considering the various types of biomarkers and their applications, it is appropriate to address the one application that may be considered 'the elephant in the room' – surrogate endpoints. The Biomarkers Definitions Working Group defined a 'surrogate endpoint' as:

'A biomarker that is intended to substitute for a clinical endpoint. A surrogate endpoint is expected to predict clinical benefit (or harm or lack of benefit or harm) based on epidemiologic, therapeutic, pathophysiologic, or other scientific evidence.' [4]

Indeed a 'clinical endpoint' is 'a characteristic or variable that reflects how a patient feels, functions, or survives' [4]. As such, clinical endpoints such as overall survival (OS, the time from randomization to death from any cause), are regarded as the most rigorous and credible measures of clinical benefit from therapeutic intervention. On the other hand, such clinical endpoints generally dictate a large study sample size and duration, and are influenced by multiple factors [19,20]. Conceptually a surrogate endpoint is an endpoint that responds to therapeutic intervention in a shorter time frame and/or with a smaller sample size than the clinical endpoint which it is substituting for. Thus a surrogate endpoint serves to accelerate the drug development and regulatory registration processes [4,21–23]. Such an application makes regulatory acceptance of a biomarker as a surrogate endpoint highly desirable, 1) to the pharmaceutical industry as a means of both reducing cost and time to market, and 2) to patient advocates as a means for bringing promising therapies into practice sooner [24]. However, an effect on a surrogate endpoint usually is not in and of itself a benefit to the patient; rather the value of a surrogate endpoint response is in its connection to a subsequent clinical outcome [25]. As one clear example of a surrogate endpoint, accepted by both clinicians and regulators, blood pressure has been convincingly shown to be associated with cardiovascular disease risk in numerous epidemiological studies. Importantly, blood pressure responds to therapeutic interventions that improve cardiovascular clinical endpoints (e.g., reduce incidence of stroke) [25]. Adding confidence to the use of blood pressure as a surrogate endpoint is its response to interventions of several different types, including calcium channel blockers, diuretics and angiotension-converting enzyme inhibitors. Such a volume of supporting data is often not available at the time a biomarker is proposed as a surrogate endpoint. Statistical approaches to confirm a biomarker as a surrogate endpoint were proposed by Prentice in 1989 [26] and continue to evolve [27], but more often than not, biomarkers are suggested for use as surrogate endpoints on the basis of correlations and mechanistic assumptions. The reliance on correlation has been called into question [28]. Recently, examples where surrogate endpoints have been used to guide clinical trials, but failed to accurately anticipate clinical outcomes [29] have led to skepticism and concern over their use [30], particularly in an accelerated drug approval process [22]. Hence, the subject of biomarkers as surrogate endpoints remains both attractive and controversial. Given the important need to develop treatments for chronic and debilitating conditions such as Alzheimer's disease and chronic obstructive pulmonary disease, the slow progression of these diseases, and the lack of satisfactory clinical endpoints [20,31], the debate over the best process for efficiently identifying a biomarker as a surrogate endpoint will certainly continue.

For the most part there are three broad areas of applications biomarkers have in both drug development and clinical practice: diagnosis, prognosis and intervention management. Diagnosis is concerned with determining the current state of the subject and the existence, extent and characteristics of any disease condition. From a temporal standpoint, diagnosis is focused on the present, and as such diagnostic biomarkers can be benchmarked against other concurrent observations. Prognosis involves a prediction of the probable course and/or outcome of a disease, or risk of future disease in an otherwise healthy individual. Both of these applications invoke elements of both time and chance, i.e., probability. The multifactorial nature of causality for most diseases makes their development from any given point in time a stochastic process [32], clouding the relationship between any given observation or factor and a diagnosis of disease at a later point in time. While prognostic biomarkers are vitally important, the elements of time and probability make their qualification and application problematic. Indeed, considerable debate and research is ongoing over the methodological and statistical approaches for qualifying predictive/prognostic biomarkers [33–37], highlighting the challenges in their application. The third application of biomarkers, intervention management, may actually be an extension of the use of diagnostic and prognostic markers, but is worth considering as distinct, as the characteristics of intervention are driven by prior diagnostic and/or prognostic tests.

Diagnostic Applications

Single and Multiplex Biomarkers

As noted, diagnosis is the determination of an existing state or its characteristics. Such 'states' could include pathobiology, disease, toxicity or adverse reaction, or exposure to an environmental agent. In clinical practice, diagnosis is usually approached in response to symptoms that a patient presents, such as fatigue or unexplained weight loss. In some cases, a single biomarker may suffice to enable the diagnosis. Thus, a blood glucose level of 200 mg/dL or higher, plus the presence of the previously mentioned symptoms, is strongly diagnostic for diabetes [38]. Similarly detection of the exotoxin produced by toxigenic strains of *Corynebacterium* using an enzyme immunoassay serves as rapid diagnosis for serious diphtheria infections [39]. In the case of heavy metals such as cadmium, exposure can be diagnosed by direct measurement of the element in urine, blood or tissue [40]. More commonly, a patient's symptoms or condition can be the result of many different etiologies; proper understanding and treatment requires 'differential diagnosis' with the use of multiple biomarkers designed to rule out one or more of these etiologies. Thus, to distinguish the three types of diabetes, tests additional to 'random' blood glucose must be conducted [38]. Similarly, elevated serum alanine aminotransferase (ALT) levels alone do not distinguish viral hepatitis from drug-induced liver injury [41–43] or that from strenuous exercise [44]. Rather multiple biomarkers, including serum bilirubin, serum aspartate aminotransferase and antibodies to viral antigen, are considered. While the assessment of multiple parameters is most often approached qualitatively [45], algorithmic approaches to formally evaluated multiple endpoints (i.e., multivariate analyses) have been explored in the past [41]. With the advent of 'omic' technologies allowing the simultaneous measurements of tens to thousands of endpoints, multivariate analysis has led to the concept of the 'signature', wherein a specific algorithmic evaluation of a defined, multiple endpoint becomes the biomarker [46]. While the use of signatures was initially controversial [47], and research into their optimal derivation continues [48–53], signatures based on mRNA expression levels have been shown to be consistent across methodologies [54] and have a functional basis to their collection [55,56]. Several mRNA-based signature assays for prognostic applications in oncology are currently commercially available, with two (MammaPrint and Oncotype Dx) having convincing data supporting their clinical benefit in predicting recurrence and aggressiveness of breast cancers [57]. While much work has been carried out in developing mRNA-based signatures, protein and metabolite based signature biomarkers have also been described [58–60]. In drug development both single and multiplex or multiple biomarkers have been used in diagnostic applications.

Patient Classification/Stratification by Current State or Stage of Disease

Key to the effective treatment of many diseases is an understanding of the current state or stage of the disease in the patient. Such stages in the overall natural history of the disease are defined by a single or combination of symptoms and/or biomarkers. Thus, the natural history of chronic hepatitis B (CHB) can be classified into four major clinical phases based on the presence of serum HBsAg (hepatitis B surface antigen), the presence of HBeAg (the extracellular form of hepatits B core antigen), levels of serum alanine aminotransferase (ALT) and HBV DNA [61]. Chronic kidney disease (CKD) is diagnosed and staged by the loss of kidney function as measured by glomerular filtration rate (GFR) [62], albeit GFR is often estimated by serum levels of other biomarkers such as serum creatinine and serum cystatin C [63]. The natural history of chronic obstructive pulmonary disease (COPD) is characterized by a variety of symptoms and, most importantly, declining lung function [64], usually measured by forced expiratory volume in one second (FEV$_1$). As with CKD, COPD has been characterized by stages such as those defined by the Global Initiative for Chronic Obstructive Lung Disease (GOLD), although other measures have been advocated, such as the BODE (body mass index, obstruction, dyspnea, and exercise capacity) index (B), degree of airflow obstruction (O) as measured by FEV$_1$, dyspnea as measured by the Medical Research Council (MRC) dyspnea scale (D), and exercise capacity (E) as measured by the six minute walking distance (6MWD) test [65]. In the case of oncology, histopathology has historically proven to be the defining standard biomarker for diagnosis of the type and stage of tumor [66], and the benchmark against which molecular approaches such as prostate-specific antigen (PSA) [67] are measured.

More often than not, clinical trials in drug development use such disease classifications to determine the included patient population. Selecting trial subjects with more serious disease states, and hence 'enriching the trial population' [13] has the potential for demonstrating convincing benefit or impact on symptoms for the test drug. Furthermore, in early stages of development a novel drug may not have a completely characterized safety profile and this approach limits exposure to only those patients who might receive the most benefit. Thus, to demonstrate the impact of sevelamer, a non-calcium-based phosphate binder, on endothelial dysfunction (as measured by flow-mediated dilation [68]) in chronic kidney disease, only stage 4 CKD patients were included. Additional biomarker criteria defining the particular disease state included the absence of diabetes and phosphate levels greater than or equal to 5.5 mg/dL [69]. Similarly, to evaluate the long-term efficacy and safety of tiotropium in COPD, subjects were chosen on the basis of FEV$_1$ to have stable, moderate-to-severe airway obstruction [70]. In the field of oncology, histopathological typing and grading have historically served as the basis for clinical trial population selection, yet measures such as PSA levels have been used [71] as inclusion criteria and one might expect more examples in the future of molecular measures used to stage tumors for clinical trial selection.

Patient Classification/Stratification by Disease Target Characteristics

Certain disease characteristics, such as tumor type, are not stage dependent and often serve as the basis for more targeted therapy. In some respects these characteristics are actually prognostic or predictive of response to a certain treatment, but may be considered diagnostic in that they represent a current and future state of the disease and a necessary target of treatment. The most recent and elegant example of this is the development of ivacaftor, a drug that improves the function of the CFTR (cystic fibrosis transmembrane conductance regulator) protein in the 4–5% of cystic fibrosis patients that specifically have the G551D mutation [72]. Clinical trials were conducted with that subgroup based upon the known *in vitro* targeted pharmacology of the drug [73]. However, the earliest efforts to make use of therapies targeted to unique disease characteristics were in oncology, where a monoclonal antibody against the human epidermal growth factor receptor 2 (HER2) protein, trastuzumab, was effective primarily in a population of women with metastatic breast cancer that expressed HER2 [74]. Other efforts targeted the Bcr-Abl tyrosine kinase in chronic myeloid leukemia (CML) with a designed inhibitor, imatinib (Gleevec) [75], albeit this drug has shown efficacy in other tumors. A number of targeted therapies are now being developed, such as gefitinib for patients with advanced non-small-cell lung cancer that are positive for mutations in epidermal growth factor receptor (EGFR) or alterations in its expression [76]. The promise of such tumor characterization leading to effective treatment has led to the I-SPY2 adaptive breast cancer trial as an effort to further broaden the repertoire of biomarkers that might stratify breast cancer [77]. The use of selection biomarkers in late stage clinical trials has been recently reviewed [78], with the observation that this application could be further developed, as some of the more common tumors, such as prostate, have yet to be explored for biomarkers that may segment the patient population. Most certainly such molecular biomarker classification is not limited to cancer, an example being the treatment of chronic heart failure with the beta-blocker bucindolol, where an alpha2C-adrenergic receptor polymorphism alters the drugs norepinephrine-lowering effects and therapeutic response [79,80].

Patient Stratification/Selection by Metabolism Characteristics

Molecular biology made one of its first impacts on drug development in the area of drug metabolism and pharmacokinetics. DNA cloning and sequencing allowed the identification and precise characterization of different drug metabolism isoenzymes (initially cytochrome P450s) from both preclinical species and humans [81]. Initially this information was used to understand the differences in pharmacokinetics between the different species used in drug development, but, as noted earlier, the molecular approach soon revealed that inter-individual differences in drug ADME and response may be linked to molecular differences in particular drug metabolizing or transporting enzymes.

One of the early examples of pharmacogenomics was the discovery that inter-individual differences in the response to 6-mercaptopurine (6MP) treatment could be tied to genetic differences in the locus for thiopurine S-methyltransferase (TPMT) [82]. Polymorphisms in this gene can result in dramatic loss of activity, abrogating the methylation and inactivation of 6MP and thioguanine. Since thiopurine therapy is a balance between tumor suppression and myelosuppression, the concentration of circulating active drug is critical. Individuals with two inactive TPMT alleles universally experience serious myelosuppression, with heterozygous individuals also being at risk for thiopurine toxicity. The relationship between the genotype and phenotype is such that guidelines have been developed for treatment based on genetic tests [83]. The TMPT genotype does not currently play a critical role in drug development, but it has created a paradigm that is guiding other pharmacogenomic approaches.

CYP2D6 was one of the first drug metabolizing liver isoenzymes to be found to vary in activity between individuals, with profound effects on anti-depressant treatments [84,85]. This enzyme is responsible for the clearance of a large percentage of drugs, and individuals characterized as 'poor metabolizers' (PM) and undergoing perhexiline treatment show adverse effects and toxicity. A large number of genetic variants are associated with the PM phenotype; in addition, gene duplications and other variations can be associated with an 'ultrarapid metabolizer' (UM) phenotype. For drugs such as tamoxifen and oxycodone analgesics, therapeutic response has been convincingly demonstrated to be affected by CYP2D6 phenotype [86,87]. Since the antitussive agent dextromethorphan (DM) is metabolized rapidly mainly through the action of CYP2D6, the levels of various DM metabolites in plasma and urine may be used to assess CYP2D6 phenotype, i.e., enzyme activity [88,89]. The correlations between CYP2D6 genetic variants and enzyme activity turn out to be good enough to allow models to be developed that can predict the pharmacokinetics of a drug like DM based on genotype [88,90] as tested with various diagnostic techniques such as the Roche AmpliChip P450 test, which tests CYP2D6 genotype in addition to that of CYP2C19 [91]. Given such background it is not surprising to find reports of clinical trials such as that of AZD3480 where, given the extensive metabolism of this investigative drug by CYP2D6, patient dosing was based upon CYP2D6 genotype [92].

As discussed above, the application of ADME pharmacogenomics across the pharmaceutical industry was examined in a 2008 white paper [9]. Of particular note here is that the 'biomarkers' of focus are indeed genetic; i.e., gene variants. While genotype biomarkers have certain advantages, the white paper notes that their determination may not always be technically trivial, and that most established genotyping technologies look for known variants and may miss novel polymorphisms. Furthermore, drugs whose ADME is suggested by preclinical studies to be dependent upon a particular Cyp enzyme may have a clinical ADME profile that is relatively insensitive to the corresponding genotype of patients. Nevertheless, a large number of pharmaceutical companies collect material in early clinical studies for follow-up genotyping if individual patient differences in ADME are suspected to be due to metabolic enzyme or transporter variants [14].

Prognostic Applications

Patient Stratification by Expected Disease Progression or Clinical Outcome

In many respects stratification by predicted disease progression or clinical outcome is similar to stratification by the stage of the disease. The distinction may be seen in that in the latter case the natural history of the disease has been reasonably established, and the understanding is that most patients at a certain stage will progress to the next stage. However, not all pathological conditions have a clearly defined natural history, or their progression to clinical outcomes differs considerably from patient to patient. In such cases a measurement that is prognostic for serious clinical outcome in a given patient, and differentiates that patient from those whose condition will not progress, will identify that patient as a candidate for therapeutic intervention. In a clinical trial setting, such 'prognostic enrichment' [13] for patients expected to have more serious outcomes without treatment will more clearly demonstrate the effectiveness of an experiment treatment.

Of course, and as noted above, the elements of time and probability make prognostic biomarkers challenging to identify and apply. Nonetheless, the importance of identifying patients most in need of treatment and of developing effective drugs for them drives continued efforts to discover and qualify prognostic biomarkers. Thus while the 'natural history' of COPD has been described, not all patients have similar rates of decline in lung function, prompting a search for plasma biomarkers that could distinguish 'rapid decliners' from 'slow decliners' [58]. If confirmed and qualified in studies with larger cohorts, such a biomarker could serve to enrich a clinical trial with patients whose disease would be impacted by effective treatment in a short time period than the overall COPD population. COPD is also complicated by exacerbations, episodic symptoms of increased cough, dyspnea and respiratory distress. These exacerbations contribute to the morbidity and burden of the disease, yet do not occur with equal frequency in all patients. Levels of plasma fibrinogen were found to be predictive of severe exacerbations, and would serve as a means to enrich a COPD patient population with those individuals most likely to benefit from a treatment that would ameliorate the disease or reduce the incidence of exacerbations [93]. Septic shock is another condition where there is broad heterogeneity in patient outcome, and where the interpretation of interventional trials is complicated by those patients whose condition resolves with minimal or standard treatment. To this end a series of serum markers, including ones indicative of apoptosis, were identified as potential early predictors for survival in severe septic patients with hepatic dysfunction [94]. Toward a similar goal, plasma interleukin-8 was examined for its ability to predict 28-day mortality in pediatric septic shock [95]. A training set was used to establish a cutoff serum IL-8 level (220 pg/mL), and that value was found to have a negative predictive value of 94% in two subsequent sets of data. In other words, use of this biomarker could exclude those patients with 95% predicted survivorship, and allow for a clinical trial population most likely to benefit from therapy. Similarly not all patients with CKD progress to dialysis and death (end stage renal disease, ESRD) at the same rate; asymmetric dimethylarginine (ADMA), a marker of atherosclerosis was found to be an independent predictor of ESRD [96], suggesting its use as a clinical trial stratification tool. Finally, both serum and urinary neutrophil gelatinase-associated lipocalin (NGAL) was found to be highly predictive early for acute renal injury after cardiac surgery, suggesting its use for selecting patients most likely to benefit from therapeutic intervention [97].

Of course, oncology represents a therapeutic area where prediction of the clinical outcome for any given patient or group of patients would have great impact on both therapy and clinical trial design. One early example is that of the seven factor score developed by Hasenclever and Diehl that predicts five year rates of freedom from progression for patients with Hodgkin's lymphoma [98]. With the advent of molecular tools, genomic investigations have been undertaken and numerous multi-gene signatures have been reported. Thus an 11-gene signature based on the BMI-1 pathway was proposed as 'death-from-cancer' signature for multiple types of cancer [99], and a 70 gene signature was reported as a predictor of multi-year disease outcome in patients with breast cancer [100]. The investigation of such prognostic gene signatures has led to commercially available tests [57,101], and the role of such prognostic biomarkers in cancer therapy has been reviewed [102].

Patient Stratification by Risk of Disease

This category of application is subtly different in that the biomarker predicts the onset of disease or disease events in otherwise asymptomatic patients. One of the oldest and most accepted example is that of diastolic blood pressure, whose elevation is predictive of stroke and coronary heart disease (CHD) events [25]. Blood markers such as C-reactive protein (CRP) appear to be predictive of risk of cardiovascular disease [103]. Prostate-specific antigen (PSA) has long been used as an early screen for prostate cancer [67], although questions have been raised regarding its value in reducing prostate cancer mortality [104]. However, a true example of a predictive marker in cancer is that of BRCA1 and BRCA2 mutations which indicate an elevated risk of breast cancer [67], albeit even though other factors clearly affect the ultimate development of disease.

Patient Stratification by Prediction of Treatment Response

Again this category may be considered to be subtly different from the others, in that the prediction is relevant to a specific drug, and not due to metabolism. Such is the case with bucindolol, a novel α2C-adrenergic receptor blocking agent (that also acts as a sympatholytic agent). Patients that carried α2C-adrenergic receptor gene polymorphisms (specifically α2C-Del carriers) responded differently to the drug yet had no evidence of a favorable survival benefit from treatment [80]. Other polymorphisms also seem to affect the pharmacodynamics of this drug [79]. Another example may be found in a recent study of perfinidone, which appears effective in only a subpopulation of patients with idiopathic pulmonary fibrosis, as determined by a combination of physiological measurements [105].

Intervention Management/Monitoring

Target Engagement/Modulation

One very active application of genomics has been the identification of new hypothetical molecular targets for drug therapy. These new tools allow the identification of such targets through, for example, genetic studies, and investigation of the molecule's role in the organism through the use of transgenic animals. Furthermore, these tools allow the rapid screening of molecules that may interact with that target. Even so, the reality of drug development is that not all carefully designed candidate drugs may actually reach, or bind to, or modulate their intended target in a clinical setting. Thus, biomarkers that can measure such target engagement can play a critical role in confirming the viability of a candidate drug [106]. Ideally such a biomarker can indicate that:

1) the drug has indeed interacted with the target,
2) the dose level needed for this interaction is below that which would produce toxicity, and
3) these dose levels are suitable for subsequent clinical studies.

A good case study example for the use of target engagement biomarkers (and biomarkers more directly related to the disease process) is that of Merck's development of sitagliptin, a novel inhibitor of plasma dipeptidyl-peptidase IV (DPP4) for type 2 diabetes treatment [107]. In this case DPP4 inhibition in plasma served as a biomarker of target engagement, levels of glucagon-like peptide-1 (GLP-1) and glucose-dependent insulinotropic peptide (GIP) served as biomarkers of target modulation, and glucose levels represented a measure of the impact of treatment on the disease. The proof-of-concept for both the molecule and mechanism of action allowed the subsequent drug development program to proceed with less risk of failure. It should also be noted that these biomarkers were operative in non-clinical studies as well.

Response Monitoring

Obviously biomarkers that monitor the state or stage of disease may be used to monitor response to therapy, assuming that they are monitoring symptoms or characteristics that are reversible. Blood pressure has long been accepted as such a biomarker and the anti-hypertensive effects of agents, such as lisinopril, that inhibit angiotensin-converting enzyme have long been recognized [108]. Relevant to monitoring response in clinical trials is the question of what response is clinically relevant, i.e., the Minimal Clinically Important Difference (MCID) [109,110]. This question is not trivial and is subject to debate. Nonetheless, the concept of MCID has served to guide several biomarker studies, such as that of the 6-minute-walk test (6MWT) as a measure of exercise tolerance in idiopathic pulmonary fibrosis (IPF) [111]. As noted above, surrogate endpoints represent the 'holy grail' in response monitoring biomarkers, but biomarkers not yet accepted as surrogate endpoints may still have great value in understanding the results of a clinical trial [112] and in estimating the size of pivotal trials from the results of exploratory studies.

Adverse Event or Toxicity Monitoring

The regulatory requirement for new drugs to be 'safe and effective' clearly mandates that safety be monitored in drug development clinical trials. Given the importance of such monitoring, the biomarkers used are generally those with considerable experience and historical data attached to them. Such is the case with monitors of drug-induced liver injury (DILI), where despite the interest in newly discovered biomarkers of hepatotoxicity [113], clinical DILI is assessed using a combination of measurements of serum transaminase and serum total bilirubin [43]. On the other hand, cardiac troponins (cTns), which are well established as measures of clinical ischemic cardiac disease, have gained considerable support as both non-clinical and clinical monitors of cardiotoxicity [114–116]. Other organ systems such as the kidney lack truly sensitive measures for monitoring toxicity, with newly developed biomarkers offering promise [117]. But in this area, as in many, an efficient process of clinical biomarker acceptance or qualification has not yet been truly established. Of course, that is the subject of the other chapters of this book.

Concluding Remarks

As noted, the uses of biomarkers in drug development have been discussed in several books and reviews; the purpose here was to present an overview that would provide perspective to the following chapters on biomarker qualification. In particular the different characteristics of diagnostic biomarker, prognostic biomarkers and surrogate endpoints impact the approaches to their acceptance and qualification. Their application in drug development and medicine in general will also be driven by not merely scientific, but also economic considerations [118,119]. It will be a combination of scientific merit, economic benefit, regulatory implication and medical impact that will move the field of biomarkers forward from a 'fad' to a cornerstone of biomedical research and health care practice.

References

[1] Dews I. Biomarkers are not new. In: Bleavins MR, Carini C, Jurima-Romet M, Rahbaria R, editors. Biomarkers in Drug Development. New Jersey: John Wiley & Sons; 2010. p. 3–14. Hoboken.

[2] Allen JP. The Art of Medicine in Ancient Egypt. Metropolitan Museum of Art 2005. New York. ISBN: 9780300107289.

[3] Eknoyan G. Looking at the urine: the renaissance of an unbroken tradition. Am J Kidney Dis 2007; 49:865–72.

[4] Biomarkers Definitions Working Group. Biomarkers and surrogate endpoints: preferred definitions and conceptual framework. Clin Pharmacol Ther 2001;69:89–95.

[5] Karpetsky TP, Humphrey RL, Levy CC. Influence of renal insufficiency on levels of serum ribonuclease in patients with multiple myeloma. J Natl Cancer Inst 1977;58:875–80.

[6] Pedersen KO. Ultracentrifugal and electrophoretic studies on fetuin. J Phys Colloid Chem 1947;51: 164–71.

[7] Kanbay M, Nicoleta M, Selcoki Y, Ikizek M, Aydin M, Eryonucu B, et al. Fibroblast growth factor 23 and fetuin A are independent predictors for the coronary artery disease extent in mild chronic kidney disease. Clin J Am Soc Nephrol 2010;5:1780–6.

[8] Mori K, Emoto M, Inaba M. Fetuin-A: a multifunctional protein. Recent Pat Endocr Metab Immune Drug Discov 2011;5:124–46.

[9] Williams JA, Andersson T, Andersson TB, Blanchard R, Behm MO, Cohen N, et al. PhRMA white paper on ADME pharmacogenomics. J Clin Pharmacol 2008;48:849–89.

[10] ICH and International Conference on Harmonization. Definitions for genomic biomarkers, pharmacogenomics, pharmacogenetics, genomic data and sample coding categories: E15. In: ICH Harmonised Tripartite Guideline Geneva, Switzerland 2007: DOC.E15-Step4.

[11] Committee For Human Medicinal Products, European Medicines Agency. Guidelines on Pharmacogenetics Briefing Meetings 2006: DOC. Ref. EMEA/CHMP/PGxWP/20227/2004.

[12] US FDA. Guidance for Industry. Clinical Pharmacogenomics: Premarketing Evaluation in Early-Phase Clinical Studies and Recommendations for Labeling. Silver Spring, MD: 2013: UCM337169. pdf.

[13] Temple R. Enrichment of clinical study populations. Clin Pharmacol Ther 2010;88:774–8.

[14] Grecco N, Cohen N, Warner AW, Lopez-Correa C, Truter SL, Snapir A, et al. PhRMA survey of pharmacogenomic and pharmacodynamic evaluations: what next? Clin Pharmacol Ther 2012;91: 1035–43.

[15] Buyse M, Michiels S, Sargent DJ, Grothey A, Matheson A, de Gramont A. Integrating biomarkers in clinical trials. Expert Rev Mol Diagn 2011;11:171–82.

[16] Sikorski R, Yao B. Parallel paths to predictive biomarkers in oncology: Uncoupling of emergent biomarker development and phase III trial execution. Sci Transl Med 2009;1:10ps11.

[17] Dancey JE, Dobbin KK, Groshen S, Jessup JM, Hruszkewycz AH, Koehler M, et al. Guidelines for the development and incorporation of biomarker studies in early clinical trials of novel agents. Clin Cancer Res 2010;16:1745–55.

[18] Mestan KK, Ilkhanoff L, Mouli S, Lin S. Genomic sequencing in clinical trials. J Transl Med 2011;9:222.

[19] Verma S, McLeod D, Batist G, Robidoux A, Martins IR, Mackey JR. In the end what matters most? A review of clinical endpoints in advanced breast cancer. Oncologist 2011;16:25–35.

[20] Glaab T, Vogelmeier C, Buhl R. Outcome measures in chronic obstructive pulmonary disease (COPD): strengths and limitations. Respir Res 2010;11:79–89.

[21] Psaty BM, Weiss NS, Furberg CD, Koepsell TD, Siscovick DS, Rosendaal FR, et al. Surrogate end points, health outcomes, and the drug-approval process for the treatment of risk factors for cardiovascular disease. Jama 1999;282:786–90.

[22] Fleming TR. Surrogate endpoints and FDA's accelerated approval process. Health Aff (Millwood) 2005;24:67–78.

[23] Park JW, Kerbel RS, Kelloff GJ, Barrett JC, Chabner BA, Parkinson DR, et al. Rationale for biomarkers and surrogate end points in mechanism-driven oncology drug development. Clin Cancer Res 2004;10:3885–96.

[24] Kelloff GJ, Bast Jr RC, Coffey DS, D'Amico AV, Kerbel RS, Park JW, et al. Biomarkers, surrogate end points, and the acceleration of drug development for cancer prevention and treatment: an update prologue. Clin Cancer Res 2004;10:3881–4.

[25] Desai M, Stockbridge N, Temple R. Blood pressure as an example of a biomarker that functions as a surrogate. Aaps J 2006;8:E146–152.

[26] Prentice RL. Surrogate endpoints in clinical trials: definition and operational criteria. Stat Med 1989;8:431–40.

[27] Buyse M, Molenberghs G, Burzykowski T, Renard D, Geys H. The validation of surrogate endpoints in meta-analyses of randomized experiments. Biostatistics 2000;1:49–67.

[28] Baker SG, Kramer BS. A perfect correlate does not a surrogate make. BMC Med Res Methodol 2003;3:16.

[29] Psaty BM, Lumley T. Surrogate end points and FDA approval: a tale of 2 lipid-altering drugs. Jama 2008;299:1474–6.

[30] Anand IS, Florea VG, Fisher L. Surrogate end points in heart failure. J Am Coll Cardiol 2002;39: 1414–21.

[31] Romero K, de Mars M, Frank D, Anthony M, Neville J, Kirby L, et al. The Coalition Against Major Diseases: developing tools for an integrated drug development process for Alzheimer's and Parkinson's diseases. Clin Pharmacol Ther 2009;86:365–7.

[32] Coggon DI, Martyn CN. Time and chance: the stochastic nature of disease causation. Lancet 2005; 365:1434–7.

[33] Cook NR. Use and misuse of the receiver operating characteristic curve in risk prediction. Circulation 2007;115:928–35.

[34] Subtil F, Pouteil-Noble C, Toussaint S, Villar E, Rabilloud M. A simple modeling-free method provides accurate estimates of sensitivity and specificity of longitudinal disease biomarkers. Methods Inf Med 2009;48:299–305.

[35] Taylor JM, Ankerst DP, Andridge RR. Validation of biomarker-based risk prediction models. Clin Cancer Res 2008;14:5977–83.

[36] Vickers AJ, Cronin AM, Elkin EB, Gonen M. Extensions to decision curve analysis, a novel method for evaluating diagnostic tests, prediction models and molecular markers. BMC Med Inform Decis Mak 2008;8:53.

[37] Cook NR. Statistical evaluation of prognostic versus diagnostic models: beyond the ROC curve. Clin Chem 2008;54:17–23.

[38] National Diabetes Information Clearinghouse. Diagnosis of diabetes, US Dept. of Health and Human Services 2008; Report No. NIH No. 09-4642.

[39] Efstratiou A, Engler KH, Mazurova IK, Glushkevich T, Vuopio-Varkila J, Popovic T. Current approaches to the laboratory diagnosis of diphtheria. J Infect Dis 2000;181(Suppl. 1):S138–145.

[40] Lu J, Jin T, Nordberg G, Nordberg M. Metallothionein gene expression in peripheral lymphocytes from cadmium-exposed workers. Cell Stress Chaperones 2001;6:97–104.

[41] Plomteux G. Multivariate analysis of an enzymic profile for the differential diagnosis of viral hepatitis. Clin Chem 1980;26:1897–9.

[42] Reichling JJ, Kaplan MM. Clinical use of serum enzymes in liver disease. Dig Dis Sci 1988;33: 1601–14.

[43] Senior JR. Drug hepatotoxicity from a regulatory perspective. Clin Liver Dis 2007;11:507–24. vi.

[44] Pettersson J, Hindorf U, Persson P, Bengtsson T, Malmqvist U, Werkstrom V, et al. Muscular exercise can cause highly pathological liver function tests in healthy men. Br J Clin Pharmacol 2008; 65:253–9.

[45] Hall RL, Everds NE. Factors affecting the interpretation of canine and nonhuman primate clinical pathology. Toxicol Pathol 2003;31(Suppl.):6–10.

[46] Segal E, Friedman N, Kaminski N, Regev A, Koller D. From signatures to models: understanding cancer using microarrays. Nat Genet 2005;37(Suppl.):S38–45.

[47] Simon R, Radmacher MD, Dobbin K, McShane LM. Pitfalls in the use of DNA microarray data for diagnostic and prognostic classification. J Natl Cancer Inst 2003;95:14–8.

[48] Kerns RT, Bushel PR. The impact of classification of interest on predictive toxicogenomics. Front Genet 2012;3:14.

[49] Rollins DK, Zhai D, Joe AL, Guidarelli JW, Murarka A, Gonzalez R. A novel data mining method to identify assay-specific signatures in functional genomic studies. BMC Bioinformatics 2006;7:377.

[50] Yang K, Cai Z, Li J, Lin G. A stable gene selection in microarray data analysis. BMC Bioinformatics 2006;7:228.

[51] Grate LR. Many accurate small-discriminatory feature subsets exist in microarray transcript data: biomarker discovery. BMC Bioinformatics 2005;6:97.

[52] Baker SG, Kramer BS. Identifying genes that contribute most to good classification in microarrays. BMC Bioinformatics 2006;7:407.

[53] Ancona N, Maglietta R, Piepoli A, D'Addabbo A, Cotugno R, Savino M, et al. On the statistical assessment of classifiers using DNA microarray data. BMC Bioinformatics 2006;7:387.

[54] Fan X, Lobenhofer EK, Chen M, Shi W, Huang J, Luo J, et al. Consistency of predictive signature genes and classifiers generated using different microarray platforms. Pharmacogenomics J 2010; 10:247–57.

[55] Shi W, Bessarabova M, Dosymbekov D, Dezso Z, Nikolskaya T, Dudoladova M, et al. Functional analysis of multiple genomic signatures demonstrates that classification algorithms choose phenotype-related genes. Pharmacogenomics J 2010;10:310–23.

[56] Bild AH, Yao G, Chang JT, Wang Q, Potti A, Chasse D, et al. Oncogenic pathway signatures in human cancers as a guide to targeted therapies. Nature 2006;439:353–7.

[57] Marchionni L, Wilson RF, Wolff AC, Marinopoulos S, Parmigiani G, Bass EB, et al. Systematic review: gene expression profiling assays in early-stage breast cancer. Ann Intern Med 2008;148:358–69.

[58] Devanarayan V, Scholand MB, Hoidal J, Leppert MF, Crackower MA, O'Neill GP, et al. Identification of distinct plasma biomarker signatures in patients with rapid and slow declining forms of COPD. Copd 2010;7:51–8.

[59] Shaham O, Slate NG, Goldberger O, Xu Q, Ramanathan A, Souza AL, et al. A plasma signature of human mitochondrial disease revealed through metabolic profiling of spent media from cultured muscle cells. Proc Natl Acad Sci U S A 2010;107:1571–5.

[60] Theodorescu D, Wittke S, Ross MM, Walden M, Conaway M, Just I, et al. Discovery and validation of new protein biomarkers for urothelial cancer: a prospective analysis. Lancet Oncol 2006;7:230–40.

[61] Lau DT, Bleibel W. Current status of antiviral therapy for hepatitis B. Therap Adv Gastroenterol 2008;1:61–75.

[62] Levey AS, Eckardt KU, Tsukamoto Y, Levin A, Coresh J, Rossert J, et al. Definition and classification of chronic kidney disease: a position statement from Kidney Disease: Improving Global Outcomes (KDIGO). Kidney Int 2005;67:2089–100.

[63] Stevens LA, Coresh J, Schmid CH, Feldman HI, Froissart M, Kusek J, et al. Estimating GFR using serum cystatin C alone and in combination with serum creatinine: a pooled analysis of 3,418 individuals with CKD. Am J Kidney Dis 2008;51:395–406.

[64] Viegi G, Pistelli F, Sherrill DL, Maio S, Baldacci S, Carrozzi L. Definition, epidemiology and natural history of COPD. Eur Respir J 2007;30:993–1013.

[65] Cote CG, Celli BR. BODE index: a new tool to stage and monitor progression of chronic obstructive pulmonary disease. Pneumonol Alergol Pol 2009;77:305–13.

[66] Cardiff RD, Gregg JP, Miller JW, Axelrod DE, Borowsky AD. Histopathology as a predictive biomarker: strengths and limitations. J Nutr 2006;136:2673S–5S.

[67] Chatterjee SK, Zetter BR. Cancer biomarkers: knowing the present and predicting the future. Future Oncol 2005;1:37–50.

[68] Kelm M. Flow-mediated dilatation in human circulation: diagnostic and therapeutic aspects. Am J Physiol Heart Circ Physiol 2002;282:H1–5.

[69] Caglar K, Yilmaz MI, Saglam M, Cakir E, Acikel C, Eyileten T, et al. Short-term treatment with sevelamer increases serum fetuin-a concentration and improves endothelial dysfunction in chronic kidney disease stage 4 patients. Clin J Am Soc Nephrol 2008;3:61–8.

[70] Bateman E, Singh D, Smith D, Disse B, Towse L, Massey D, et al. Efficacy and safety of tiotropium Respimat SMI in COPD in two 1-year randomized studies. Int J Chron Obstruct Pulmon Dis 2010;5:197–208.

[71] Morant R, Bernhard J, Dietrich D, Gillessen S, Bonomo M, Borner M, et al. Capecitabine in hormone-resistant metastatic prostatic carcinoma – a phase II trial. Br J Cancer 2004;90:1312–7.

[72] Accurso FJ, Rowe SM, Clancy JP, Boyle MP, Dunitz JM, Durie PR, et al. Effect of VX-770 in persons with cystic fibrosis and the G551D-CFTR mutation. N Engl J Med 2010;363:1991–2003.

[73] Van Goor F, Hadida S, Grootenhuis PD, Burton B, Cao D, Neuberger T, et al. Rescue of CF airway epithelial cell function in vitro by a CFTR potentiator, VX-770. Proc Natl Acad Sci U S A 2009;106:18825–30.

[74] Lee CK, Lord SJ, Coates AS, Simes RJ. Molecular biomarkers to individualise treatment: assessing the evidence. Med J Aust 2009;190:631–6.

[75] Druker BJ. Inhibition of the Bcr-Abl tyrosine kinase as a therapeutic strategy for CML. Oncogene 2002;21:8541–6.

[76] Pennell NA, Sequist LV. Assessing the roles of EGFR gene copy number, protein expression and mutation in predicting outcomes in non-small-cell lung cancer after treatment with EGFR inhibitors. Biomarkers Med 2007;1:203–7.

[77] Barker AD, Sigman CC, Kelloff GJ, Hylton NM, Berry DA, Esserman LJ. I-SPY 2: an adaptive breast cancer trial design in the setting of neoadjuvant chemotherapy. Clin Pharmacol Ther 2009;86:97–100.

[78] Sikorski R, Yao B. Visualizing the landscape of selection biomarkers in current phase III oncology clinical trials. Sci Transl Med 2010;2. 34ps27.

[79] Smart NA, Kwok N, Holland DJ, Jayasighe R, Giallauria F. Bucindolol: a pharmacogenomic perspective on its use in chronic heart failure. Clin Med Insights Cardiol 2011;5:55–66.

[80] Bristow MR, Murphy GA, Krause-Steinrauf H, Anderson JL, Carlquist JF, Thaneemit-Chen S, et al. An alpha2C-adrenergic receptor polymorphism alters the norepinephrine-lowering effects and therapeutic response of the beta-blocker bucindolol in chronic heart failure. Circ Heart Fail 2010;3:21–8.

[81] Gonzalez FJ. The molecular biology of cytochrome P450s. Pharmacol Rev 1988;40:243–88.

[82] Weinshilboum RM. Pharmacogenomics: catechol O-methyltransferase to thiopurine S-methyltransferase. Cell Mol Neurobiol 2006;26:539–61.

[83] Relling MV, Gardner EE, Sandborn WJ, Schmiegelow K, Pui CH, Yee SW, et al. Clinical pharmacogenetics implementation consortium guidelines for thiopurine methyltransferase genotype and thiopurine dosing. Clin Pharmacol Ther 2011;89:387–91.

[84] Lobello KW, Preskorn SH, Guico-Pabia CJ, Jiang Q, Paul J, Nichols AI, et al. Cytochrome P450 2D6 phenotype predicts antidepressant efficacy of venlafaxine: a secondary analysis of 4 studies in major depressive disorder. J Clin Psychiatry 2010;71:1482–7.

[85] Gardiner SJ, Begg EJ. Pharmacogenetics, drug-metabolizing enzymes, and clinical practice. Pharmacol Rev 2006;58:521–90.

[86] Samer CF, Daali Y, Wagner M, Hopfgartner G, Eap CB, Rebsamen MC, et al. Genetic polymorphisms and drug interactions modulating CYP2D6 and CYP3A activities have a major effect on oxycodone analgesic efficacy and safety. Br J Pharmacol 2010;160:919–30.

[87] Goetz MP, Kamal A, Ames MM. Tamoxifen pharmacogenomics: the role of CYP2D6 as a predictor of drug response. Clin Pharmacol Ther 2008;83:160–6.

[88] Abduljalil K, Frank D, Gaedigk A, Klaassen T, Tomalik-Scharte D, Jetter A, et al. Assessment of activity levels for CYP2D6*1, CYP2D6*2, and CYP2D6*41 genes by population pharmacokinetics of dextromethorphan. Clin Pharmacol Ther 2010;88:643–51.

[89] de Graan AJ, Teunissen SF, de Vos FY, Loos WJ, van Schaik RH, de Jongh FE, et al. Dextromethorphan as a phenotyping test to predict endoxifen exposure in patients on tamoxifen treatment. J Clin Oncol 2011;29:3240–6.

[90] Tod M, Goutelle S, Gagnieu MC. Genotype-based quantitative prediction of drug exposure for drugs metabolized by CYP2D6. Clin Pharmacol Ther 2011;90:582–7.

[91] de Leon J, Susce MT, Johnson M, Hardin M, Maw L, Shao A, et al. DNA microarray technology in the clinical environment: the AmpliChip CYP450 test for CYP2D6 and CYP2C19 genotyping. CNS Spectr 2009;14:19–34.

[92] Velligan D, Brenner R, Sicuro F, Walling D, Riesenberg R, Sfera A, et al. Assessment of the effects of AZD3480 on cognitive function in patients with schizophrenia. Schizophr Res 2012;134:59–64.

[93] Groenewegen KH, Postma DS, Hop WC, Wielders PL, Schlosser NJ, Wouters EF. Increased systemic inflammation is a risk factor for COPD exacerbations. Chest 2008;133:350–7.

[94] Hofer S, Brenner T, Bopp C, Steppan J, Lichtenstern C, Weitz J, et al. Cell death serum biomarkers are early predictors for survival in severe septic patients with hepatic dysfunction. Crit Care 2009;13:R93.

[95] Wong HR, Cvijanovich N, Wheeler DS, Bigham MT, Monaco M, Odoms K, et al. Interleukin-8 as a stratification tool for interventional trials involving pediatric septic shock. Am J Respir Crit Care Med 2008;178:276–82.

[96] Ravani P, Tripepi G, Malberti F, Testa S, Mallamaci F, Zoccali C. Asymmetrical dimethylarginine predicts progression to dialysis and death in patients with chronic kidney disease: a competing risks modeling approach. J Am Soc Nephrol 2005;16:2449–55.

[97] Mishra J, Dent C, Tarabishi R, Mitsnefes MM, Ma Q, Kelly C, et al. Neutrophil gelatinase-associated lipocalin (NGAL) as a biomarker for acute renal injury after cardiac surgery. Lancet 2005;365:1231–8.

[98] Hasenclever D, Diehl V. A prognostic score for advanced Hodgkin's disease. International Prognostic Factors Project on Advanced Hodgkin's Disease. N Engl J Med 1998;339:1506–14.

[99] Glinsky GV, Berezovska O, Glinskii AB. Microarray analysis identifies a death-from-cancer signature predicting therapy failure in patients with multiple types of cancer. J Clin Invest 2005;115:1503–21.

[100] van de Vijver MJ, He YD, van't Veer LJ, Dai H, Hart AA, Voskuil DW, et al. A gene-expression signature as a predictor of survival in breast cancer. N Engl J Med 2002;347:1999–2009.

[101] Ross JS, Hatzis C, Symmans WF, Pusztai L, Hortobagyi GN. Commercialized multigene predictors of clinical outcome for breast cancer. Oncologist 2008;13:477–93.

[102] Lord S, Lee C, Simes RJ. The Role of Prognostic and Predictive Markers in Cancer. Cancer Forum 2008;32:139–42.

[103] Gonzalez MA, Selwyn AP. Endothelial function, inflammation, and prognosis in cardiovascular disease. Am J Med 2003;115(Suppl. 8A):99S–106S.

[104] Lin K, Croswell JM, Koenig H, Lam C, Maltz A. Prostate-Specific Antigen-Based Screening for Prostate Cancer: An Evidence Update for the US Preventive Services Task Force. US Dept. of Health and Human Services (Agency for Healthcare Research) 2011: Report No.: 12-05160-EF-1.

[105] Azuma A, Taguchi Y, Ogura T, Ebina M, Taniguchi H, Kondoh Y, et al. Exploratory analysis of a phase III trial of pirfenidone identifies a subpopulation of patients with idiopathic pulmonary fibrosis as benefiting from treatment. Respir Res 2011;12:143.

[106] Frank R, Hargreaves R. Clinical biomarkers in drug discovery and development. Nat Rev Drug Discov 2003;2:566–80.

[107] Krishna R, Herman G, Wagner JA. Accelerating drug development using biomarkers: a case study with sitagliptin, a novel DPP4 inhibitor for type 2 diabetes. Aaps J 2008;10:401–9.

[108] Noble TA, Murray KM. Lisinopril: a nonsulfhydryl angiotensin-converting enzyme inhibitor. Clin Pharm 1988;7:659–69.

[109] Rennard SI. Minimal clinically important difference, clinical perspective: an opinion. Copd 2005;2:51–5.

[110] Kvien TK, Heiberg T, Hagen KB. Minimal clinically important improvement/difference (MCII/ MCID) and patient acceptable symptom state (PASS): what do these concepts mean? Ann Rheum Dis 2007;66(Suppl. 3):iii40–41.

[111] Bois RM, Weycker D, Albera C, Bradford WZ, Costabel U, Kartashov A, et al. Six-minute-walk test in idiopathic pulmonary fibrosis: test validation and minimal clinically important difference. Am J Respir Crit Care Med 2011;183:1231–7.

[112] Cazzola M, MacNee W, Martinez FJ, Rabe KF, Franciosi LG, Barnes PJ, et al. Outcomes for COPD pharmacological trials: from lung function to biomarkers. Eur Respir J 2008;31:416–69.

[113] Antoine DJ, Mercer AE, Williams DP, Park BK. Mechanism-based bioanalysis and biomarkers for hepatic chemical stress. Xenobiotica 2009;39:565–77.

[114] Berridge BR, Pettit S, Walker DB, Jaffe AS, Schultze AE, Herman E, et al. A translational approach to detecting drug-induced cardiac injury with cardiac troponins: consensus and recommendations from the Cardiac Troponins Biomarker Working Group of the Health and Environmental Sciences Institute. Am Heart J 2009;158:21–9.

[115] Wallace KB, Hausner E, Herman E, Holt GD, MacGregor JT, Metz AL, et al. Serum troponins as biomarkers of drug-induced cardiac toxicity. Toxicol Pathol 2004;32:106–21.

[116] O'Brien PJ. Cardiac troponin is the most effective translational safety biomarker for myocardial injury in cardiotoxicity. Toxicology 2008;245:206–18.

[117] Dieterle F, Marrer E, Suzuki E, Grenet O, Cordier A, Vonderscher J. Monitoring kidney safety in drug development: emerging technologies and their implications. Curr Opin Drug Discov Devel 2008;11:60–71.

[118] Trusheim MR, Burgess B, Hu SX, Long T, Averbuch SD, Flynn AA, et al. Quantifying factors for the success of stratified medicine. Nat Rev Drug Discov 2011;10:817–33.

[119] Trusheim MR, Berndt ER, Douglas FL. Stratified medicine: strategic and economic implications of combining drugs and clinical biomarkers. Nat Rev Drug Discov 2007;6:287–93.

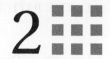

2

Impact of Biomarker Qualification Regulatory Processes on the Critical Path for Drug Development

Federico Goodsaid

STRATEGIC REGULATORY INTELLIGENCE, REGULATORY AFFAIRS, VERTEX PHARMACEUTICALS, WASHINGTON DC, USA

Introduction

A broad range of perspectives in this book describe how a complex regulatory process for biomarker qualification has been developed at regulatory agencies over the past decade. This process has now been used by the pharmaceutical industry for the past few years, and we can now take stock of its impact on pharmaceutical product development:

1) Has the process at the US Food and Drug Administration (FDA) Center for Drug Evaluation and Research (CDER) achieved the goals originally proposed by the Pharmacogenomics Guidance in 2005 [1] and the Critical Path Opportunities List and Report in 2006 [2]?
2) What are the strengths and weaknesses of the different versions of a biomarker qualification process developed in each International Committee for Harmonization (ICH) region?
3) How well have the different versions of this process been harmonized across these regions?
4) What are the opportunities and challenges for a single, universal, biomarker qualification process?
5) How can we develop metrics with which we can measure the impact of these processes on drug development and their acceptance by the pharmaceutical industry?

Not all of these questions can be addressed comprehensively with the information publicly available at this time, but a healthy discussion about the opportunities and challenges of biomarker qualification may be started with what we know thus far.

The Path from Biomarker Discovery to Regulatory Qualification. http://dx.doi.org/10.1016/B978-0-12-391496-5.00002-8

Has the Process at the FDA (CDER) Achieved the Goals Originally Proposed by the Pharmacogenomics Guidance in 2005 and the Critical Path Opportunities List and Report in 2006?

At the FDA, the immediate regulatory documentation leading to the Biomarker Qualification Process may be traced back to the Pharmacogenomics Guidance and the Critical Path Opportunities list. The Pharmacogenomics Guidance defined:

> **Valid biomarker:** *A biomarker that is measured in an analytical test system with well-established performance characteristics and for which there is an established scientific framework or body of evidence that elucidates the physiologic, toxicologic, pharmacologic, or clinical significance of the test results. The classification of biomarkers is context specific.*

There are two main challenges with this definition: the evidentiary standards which would need to be drafted to support them, and the process which would determine the validity of a biomarker. It is straightforward to establish technical specifications for a valid biomarker to be measured *in an analytical test system with well-established performance characteristics,* but how do we know that a biomarker has *an established scientific framework or body of evidence*? What makes a scientific framework or body of evidence 'established'? This definition for the standards of evidence is difficult to translate into viable metrics and to translate these viable metrics into a regulatory decision about the validity of a biomarker. A well-trodden path in the past has been to have biomarkers accepted as 'valid' not necessarily on the basis of specific standards of evidence, but on the basis of periods of public debate about their validity so long and exhausting that a final decision was often made decades later by the viability of the scientists and clinicians who survived these debates. Even after this exhausting process, critical questions about the application of accepted biomarkers may still remain incompletely addressed. A long process for acceptance through exhaustion also generates along the way a steady stream of biases which carry over to the final context of use for the biomarker.

The Guidance introduced a concept in this definition which allowed for a different discussion about how to accept biomarkers. The definition added the statement: '*The classification of biomarkers is context specific*'. While the Guidance itself referred to 'valid biomarkers' with additional subclassifications of 'known valid' and 'probable valid', the introduction of the concept of *context of use* opened a different discussion about how to accept biomarkers. If the determination of the validity of a biomarker is contingent on its context of use, then a biomarker need not be accepted as a 'valid', but rather, as 'qualified for a specific context of use'.

The context of use in biomarker qualification is a concept antithetical to the notion that a single, definitive validation is possible for a biomarker. The context of use of a biomarker aligns with the available data on the basis of how the biomarker is to be used, and not on the perceived quality of the data, which some authors have proposed as a potential classification [3] for 'validated' biomarkers. Biomarker qualification in this case is driven by the data available to support a specific context of use for the biomarker, rather than by a definitive assessment about the size or quality of the database available to evaluate a biomarker for all plausible contexts of use. This is an incremental concept, where the context of use for a biomarker expands as additional data are available: there is no definitive and universal context of use. A biomarker qualification driven by its context of use is also inconsistent with the Institute of Medicine Report [4] proposal for a single, definitive validation for biomarkers.

The introduction of the concept of 'qualification', and its contrast with the concept of 'validity' transformed the discussion about regulatory acceptance of biomarkers. A regulatory process for biomarker acceptance is viable if its goal has a finite set of evidentiary standards and a finite review cycle span. Biomarker validation is, by definition, an open-ended process with open-ended evidentiary standards, where every potential application of the biomarker needs to be supported by independent studies and datasets. Biomarker qualification, however, is a finite process with finite evidentiary standards, because for this concept a finite context of use needs to be justified by finite datasets.

Context of use is a critical concept in biomarker qualification, because it is the basic metric against which evidentiary standards need to be defined. This is clear from the perspective of the clinical or nonclinical data needed to support the qualification of a biomarker. The decades-long processes for biomarker validation often examined every conceivable scenario for the application of a biomarker, requiring also every conceivable dataset to support its use. However, if the context of use of a biomarker is circumscribed to a specific application, the datasets needed to support this application will also be circumscribed to specific, well-designed studies from which these datasets may be generated. A broad context of use for a biomarker requires (a) a clear question, (b) a scientific body of evidence, and (c) a concurrent scientific consensus, which often prevent a swift and effective application of biomarkers in drug development. Narrowing the context of the application of a biomarker facilitates its acceptance and application. For example, the application of biomarkers to better understand mechanisms of safety or efficacy is likely to require straightforward scientific evidence for a number of examples of compounds or studies justifying the mechanistic conclusions. At the other extreme, the acceptance of the application of the same biomarkers for surrogate testing may be expected to include a comprehensive evidence database across multiple compounds and studies, with thorough analytical and biological support for the proposed replacement of a pre-existing clinical endpoint.

While analytical validity may be measured through its own independent objective metrics, it is also subject to the context of use of a biomarker. For example, a specific context of use for a biomarker may require an analytical specification range for its measurement which is only a subset of the global analytical specification range available for this measurement. This prescribed range can facilitate the design of measurement platforms for this biomarker.

The process which would determine the validity of a biomarker is a separate challenge: who would determine that a biomarker is valid? As long as the decision was made through a drawn-out, exhausting public debate process, it is likely that most stakeholders in this process would also have an opportunity to participate in it. However, if a process is to be developed to review the scientific and clinical evidence supporting the validity of a biomarker, an owner for this process would need to be identified. While we have discussed here evidentiary standards and the process itself as two independent challenges, the Guidance also implied that a replacement for a decades-long process would require a consensus reached through pre-competitive collaborations by interested stakeholders organized into consortia which would supply datasets to support a qualification. The Pharmacogenomics Guidance itself did not dwell on this, but soon after this Guidance was issued, the context of use lead to a discussion [5] about who would determine that a biomarker is qualified for use in a specific context. Someone would need to determine that a biomarker is *fit for purpose*.

An initial FDA path for expert internal review in a preclinical biomarker of toxicity qualification process map [6] was tested through the Preclinical Toxicology Coordinating Committee (PTCC) with the technical assistance of the Genomics Team. In this path, the PTCC would be responsible for both the review and approval of qualification study protocols and final qualification study results. If approved by the PTCC, next steps in this process would lead to:

1) biomarker listed as probable valid, or
2) additional studies encouraged or planned to reach known valid biomarker status.

Different areas within the FDA would provide the required expert internal review for genomic biomarkers in each area. Initial steps in a qualification process such as this could be started through a Voluntary eXploratory Data Submission (VXDS), where exploratory data could be discussed and debated and preliminary validation requirements may be identified. The outcome for VXDS submissions of exploratory data in this context could range from an exciting scientific exchange about the analytical and biological interpretations of the data to the basis for additional work leading to the qualification of biomarkers.

Limitations in the original assumptions of this process map proposal were quickly identified. These were associated with the number of biomarkers, tissue toxicity models, positive and negative compounds, and other resources available to any one sponsor for qualification studies of biomarkers. These limitations underscored the need for collaboration across therapeutic areas and companies in the identification and qualification of biomarkers of toxicity.

The Critical Path Opportunities List and Report, issued in 2006, explicitly described the need for a qualification process [2]. The Critical Path Opportunities List also outlined activities started during that first year in this area:

1) Develop a concept paper on biomarker qualification.
2) Qualify oncology Biomarkers.

3) Biomarker development and qualification.
4) Predictive safety testing.
5) Predict drug effects on kidney function.

These six activities comprehensively summarize the effort at CDER over the past 6 years to develop a biomarker qualification process. A *Process Map Proposal* in 2006 [7] was one of several papers which eventually led to the draft Guidance in 2010 on the Qualification of Drug Development Tools [8]. *Biomarker Development and Qualification* led to the Pilot Process for Biomarker Qualification (2006–2009) [9]. *Qualify Oncology Biomarkers* and *Predictive Safety Testing* respectively led to the first clinical (Biomarkers Consortium [10]) and nonclinically-focused (C-Path Institute/Predictive Safety Testing Consortium [11]) biomarker qualification consortia. Biomarker data shared with the FDA as part of *Predict Drug Effects on Kidney Function* formed the core dataset for the first submission (2007) [12] and first qualification (2008) [13] in the Pilot Process for Biomarker Qualification.

The Guidance on the Qualification of Drug Development Tools [8] summarized the experience gained from each of these concepts and activities associated with the Pilot Process for Biomarker Qualification. This Guidance also supported a long-term concept for a qualification process which has been under development since the draft version of this Guidance was published. The resulting Biomarker Qualification Process captured the need shown in the Pilot Process for a Consultation and Advice period previous to a qualification submission review throughout which a submitter would be able to reach agreement with CDER reviewers on the context of use and evidentiary standards needed for qualification. In the absence of guidance on context of use determination and evidentiary standards assessment, this Consultation and Advice stage is essential for a viable Biomarker Qualification Process. This Consultation and Advice stage is followed by a data review process which closely follows what would be expected in a New Drug Application (NDA) review. A Consultation and Advice stage will not be needed once guidance is issued by CDER on Evidentiary Standards in Biomarker Qualification.

How well has this Biomarker Qualification Process fulfilled what the Pharmacogenomics Guidance and the Critical Path Opportunities List proposed? The development of the concept behind the Process itself has transformed the perspective about what is possible within a regulatory framework to introduce novel biomarkers in drug development. It has changed the popular view of a heterogeneous and unpredictable review landscape for the acceptance of new biomarkers as experienced through NDA reviews into a process and evidentiary standards which could be integrated into the critical path for drug development.

The rendering of this concept and this Process is yet to deliver on what the Guidance and the Critical Path Opportunities List promised. As of October 2012, the Biomarker Qualification Program web page [14] showed three completed biomarker qualifications. The table in this web page shows that the process yield is of about one qualification review completed every other year over the course of the six years since the Pilot Process for Biomarker Qualification was started in 2006. The Biomarker Qualification Program web page does not provide information about the cycle time for each qualification, and it also does not provide information about the number of ongoing qualifications in the Program.

However, the web page for the Biomarker Qualification Process does outline the Process as reflected in the draft Qualification Guidance for Drug Development Tools [8]. This is a slow process. The complexity and number of steps in this Process represent difficult burdens to overcome for a pre-competitive collaboration leading to a biomarker qualification. The Process includes a Pre-Submission Stage where a 'pre-review' review requires an assessment by CDER of the scientific readiness of the submission. Feedback in the Consultation and Advice stage requires a total of 16 steps. The Review stage essentially mirrors an NDA review, and adds another five steps to the Process. The Pre-Submission and Consultation and Advice stages together overshadow the length and complexity of the Review stage. While this Process accounts for critical checkpoints for qualification data, it seems counterintuitive, and contrary to the original goal of biomarker qualification, that drug approval would take a shorter time than biomarker qualification. This Process is difficult to integrate with critical path product development planning and to sell within pharmaceutical companies.

The experience available thus far in this Process could be used to accelerate its performance by drafting a guidance outlining evidentiary standards expected for a biomarker qualification submission. Knowledge by a submitter about the evidentiary standards expected would obviate the need for the Consultation and Advice stage in the Process. A direct access to regulatory review of biomarker qualification submissions could reduce the total number of steps and time needed to reach a decision.

What are the Strengths and Weaknesses of the Different Versions of a Biomarker Qualification Process Developed in Each ICH Region?

The value of similar paths for biomarker qualification in different regulatory agencies is clear. Biomarker qualification processes have been developed in regulatory agencies in the US, Europe, and Japan (FDA, EMA, and PMDA). These processes share similar scope and goals, but differ considerably in complexity and cost. Table 2.1 summarizes information on similarities and differences between these processes. This table shows the shared scope of these processes: all of these processes result in a regulatory decision. While conventional wisdom in this area has been that a regulatory process could not be developed for biomarker qualification, all three agencies have shown it can not only be developed but replicated with some characteristics unique to each agency across multiple regulatory agencies.

Process goals are also shared across all of these agencies. Scientific development and the identification of novel biomarkers are both goals which predate the development of biomarker qualification processes. Stakeholder development derives from the acknowledgment that data submission for biomarker qualification is only possible with multiple

Table 2.1   Biomarker Qualification Processes for Regulatory Agencies in the ICH Regions

Agency	FDA	EMA	PMDA
Pilot Process Start	2006	2007	2009
Scope	Regulatory Process	Regulatory Process	Regulatory Process
Goals	scientific development identification of novel biomarkers support stakeholders in development regulatory acceptance integration in regulatory review	scientific development identification of novel biomarkers support stakeholders in development regulatory acceptance integration in regulatory review	scientific development identification of novel biomarkers support stakeholders in development regulatory acceptance integration in regulatory review
Fees	0	approx. $100,000	approx. $30,000
Review Team	Shared	Shared	Shared
Minimum Number of Steps	24	12	11
Approx. Minimum Time to Decision	24 months	6 months	6 months
Qualification Decisions	3	6	1

consortia developed by stakeholders from academic, industrial and government scientists and clinicians which are actively encouraged and supported by regulatory agencies. Regulatory acceptance and integration in regulatory review are the ultimate goals of these processes. They are the most difficult to achieve, both because of the effort needed to generate, analyze, interpret, collate and submit the data as well as the effort needed to review it. The burden to generate the data for biomarker qualification and that to review it are inexorably linked because the success of all biomarker qualification efforts developed thus far by regulatory agencies is closely linked to the willingness of scientists and clinicians primarily in the pharmaceutical industry to collaborate in this process. Will regulatory reviewers throughout different agencies also accept and actively apply the results of these qualifications in their review work?

Another characteristic shared by all of these biomarker qualification processes is the shared review responsibilities for these reviewers. FDA, EMA and PMDA biomarker qualification reviewers are all recruited from relevant review divisions within each agency. This is an advantage for the rapid integration of novel biomarker qualification decisions in regulatory review, since these reviewers are closely associated with and aware of the data and interpretation which support each qualification review. However, this represents a logistical handicap for biomarker qualification review, since these reviewers will likely need to prioritize biomarker qualification activities below their main review responsibilities within each review division. It is also a source for delays above and beyond the minimum time required for a qualification decision in each agency. We would expect that, if explicit PDUFA-model funding exists for the process, along with associated timelines, priority conflicts could be addressed.

There are also major differences between these processes. The first is submission costs. While the process at the FDA is still outside of the fee structure negotiated in PDUFA V, those at the EMA and PMDA share their fee structures with scientific advice in each agency. Submission fees of approx. $100,000 at the EMA and $30,000 at the PMDA do not represent a major hurdle for consortia predominantly assembled from large pharmaceutical companies, but could represent, even at a reduced level, hurdles for consortia assembled from predominantly academic organizations or from small, startup companies.

A second, far greater hurdle in each of these processes is their complexity and length. The minimum number of steps in these processes ranges from 11 at the PMDA to 24 at the FDA, and the minimum time to a qualification decision from six months at the PMDA and EMA to 24 at the FDA. Fees may provide for shorter and predictable biomarker qualification processes, but the absence of guidance on evidentiary standards for biomarker qualification is still compensated for by long and cumbersome stages in these processes in order to reach a consensus on the datasets expected for qualification. This is a problem for consortia, because consortia membership changes within timelines often shorter than those required for the qualification process, and so does the financial support from individual members of these consortia for additional studies requested by the biomarker qualification teams in each agency. Consortium resolve wavers, and qualification efforts remain unfinished.

We do not have a published record of the number of submissions to each of these biomarker qualification processes. We do know that the number of qualification decisions thus far in all of them is limited in number and biomarker type [14]. No clear conclusions about the efficiency of each of these processes may be reached at this time, but Fig. 2.1 shows how the biomarker qualification process time could impact the outcome of a biomarkers qualification process. Human and financial resources within individual companies and consortia are finite: if the time and resources required to complete a biomarker qualification process exceed those available from individual companies and consortia, a biomarker qualification process gap (Fig. 2.1A) will result. A biomarker qualification process gap is the gap between the time and resources required by regulatory agencies for a qualification and the time and resources available for a submitter to complete a qualification. We can identify two cases where, even if time or resources are in limited supply, this biomarker qualification gap may conceivably be bridged (Fig. 2.1B):

1) Submission for qualification of a biomarker surrogate by a wide-ranging consortium of academic, government, industry and regulatory agency scientists, clinicians and patient advocates. In this case, the urgent need for a biomarker to accelerate development of critically needed therapies leads to its acceptance. A comprehensive consensus of all stakeholders interested in a surrogate is a powerful driver for qualification.

(A)

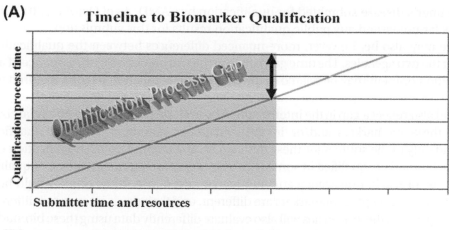

(B)

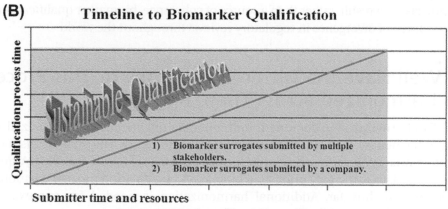

FIGURE 2.1 Timeline to biomarker qualification

2) Submission for qualification of a biomarker surrogate by a company or patient advocacy group which anticipates the need for regulatory acceptance of a surrogate preceding the anticipated submission of data supporting an NDA. This is a case where a biomarker qualification process gap is likely to be bridged, because the added value of regulatory acceptance exceeds the time and resources required to complete the biomarker qualification process.

Most biomarker qualification process gaps are not bridgeable, because the resources and time available to most consortia may not match the resources and time required to complete a biomarker qualification process.

An interesting case reflecting differences between the biomarker qualification processes developed by different regulatory agencies is shown by the submissions to the FDA and EMA [15] in 2008 for qualification from the Coalition Against Major Diseases (CAMD) [16], a Critical Path Institute Consortium, of biomarkers for Alzheimer's Disease [17]. Throughout 2011 and 2012, the EMA adopted [18,19] four qualification opinions for different biomarkers of Alzheimer's disease submitted for qualification by CAMD. As of October, 2012, the FDA has thus far not issued any public qualification results for this submission.

There may also be, however, more nuanced differences between the qualification processes at the two agencies. The time gap between the two processes in the issuance of a public qualification opinion may be related to differences in the inherent lengths required to complete the consultation and advice and review stages at the FDA and EMA. However, this time gap could also reflect a gap in the interpretation by each agency about the potential context of use for these biomarkers and/or in the evidentiary standards for these qualifications. Independently of the sources for these differences, an outcome from a qualification effort of the same biomarkers qualified in some regulatory agencies but not in others, or qualified for one context of use in one agency and another context of use in the other, would be counterproductive. If accepted biomarkers are different, or if their use is interpreted differently by different agencies, these agencies will also evaluate differently data using these biomarkers for drug approvals. As a result, rather than a source of coherence, biomarker qualification would become a source of divergence in regulatory reviews throughout the world.

How Well Have the Different Versions of This Process Been Harmonized across These Regions?

The ICH E16 harmonization document for biomarker qualification was finalized in 2010 [20] and published by the FDA, EMA and PMDA in 2011 [21]. The goal of this harmonization effort was a common submission format for the FDA, EMA and PMDA qualification processes. This is the only published biomarker qualification process harmonization document issued thus far. Additional harmonization is needed for contexts of use, evidentiary standards, and the process itself.

What are the Opportunities and Challenges for a Single, Universal, Biomarker Qualification Process?

An expansion of the content and context of the ICH E16 document would complete the harmonization of biomarker qualification at the FDA, EMA and PMDA. A harmonized biomarker qualification would add to the harmonized submission harmonized contexts of use, evidentiary standards and process. Once this level of harmonization is reached, regulatory agencies could consider a proposal for the foundation of an independent International Biomarker Qualification Center (IBQC). An IBQC would have:

1) A core staff.
2) Dedicated virtual Biomarker Qualification Review Teams (BQRT) recruited from throughout the ICH regions.
3) BQRT reviewers may include regulatory reviewers and academic and government scientists and clinicians on one year detail duty.

4) BQRT operations would be funded by a sliding fee scale for qualification submissions.

5) Public qualification decisions would be issued within a year of submissions, with a context of use pegged to the evidentiary content submitted.

6) BQRTs would expire at the end of each review cycle.

7) The legal framework for reviewer recruitment and for enforcement of IBQC BQRT decisions would be concurrently developed in all ICH regions.

8) IBQC BQRT decisions would be final and immediately implemented in all of these regions.

A good precedent for this proposal is the European Reference Laboratory on Alternatives to Animal Testing (EURL ECVAM) [22]. EURL ECVAM started in Europe in 1991 to actively support the development, validation and acceptance of methods which could reduce, refine or replace the use of laboratory animals. While the goal of this centralized test validation lab is not biomarker qualification, its international model could be adopted by a centralized biomarker qualification center.

There are, of course, major challenges in this proposal. The most difficult hurdle for a proposal like this is likely to be the legal framework needed for the US, Europe and Japan. This framework will require multiple multilateral agreements in order to succeed. However, the experience gained from harmonization attempts for biomarker qualification processes independently developed by each of these regulatory agencies suggests that the review process itself is the most critical component for the success of regulatory qualification. While other aspects of biomarker qualification may be expected to be harmonized through an expanded ICH E16 document, the review process remains the most difficult harmonization task, as it is closely aligned with other regulatory review processes in each agency. A multilateral agreement to allow for the establishment and funding of an independent IBQC would definitely be worth the effort.

How Can We Develop Metrics with Which to Measure the Impact of These Processes on Drug Development and Their Acceptance by the Pharmaceutical Industry?

One of the current major weaknesses in biomarker qualification is the paucity of data on the performance of biomarker qualification processes. Metrics to assess the success of biomarker qualification require data from both the regulatory agencies which review qualification data as well as from the companies which generate qualification data. There are several parameters which may be proposed as performance metrics for tracking the performance of a biomarker qualification process. Some should be available from regulatory agencies:

1) Total number of submissions into the process.

2) Number of submissions in each of the steps of the process.

3) Ratio of total approvals to total submissions in the process.

4) Ratio of approvals to submissions in each year.

5) Total Futility: ratio of all submissions removed from the process to total approvals.
6) Annual Futility: ratio of removals to approvals in each year.
7) Total time to a qualification decision.
8) Dwell time in each qualification process step.
9) Total time to futility for submissions removed from the process.
10) Annual time to futility for submissions removed from the process.
11) Clinical/nonclinical area breakdown for 1–10.

Other process performance parameters should be provided by submitters:

1) Company/consortium.
2) If consortium: dues and prospective study cost.
3) Total submissions.
4) Clinical/nonclinical area breakdown.
5) Regulatory agencies.
6) Rationale for submission.
7) Anticipated development phase impact.
8) Functional area origin within company.
9) Project support period within company.
10) Project support period within consortium.
11) When did test become commercially available (before, during, or after qualification process)?
12) Internal impact on biomarker discovery and development within company.

An academic interest in these parameters is no doubt overshadowed by the urgent need to address challenges in the development of biomarker qualification processes. These data need to be available internally within each regulatory agency with a biomarker qualification process, and should also be shared with current and potential biomarker qualification submitters.

Summary

Biomarker qualification regulatory processes have transformed not only the biomarker tools that we have, but the way we will use them in drug development. The concept of biomarker qualification has become integrated within that of drug development. However, the application in drug development of the processes themselves is lagging, because the complexity, time and cost required by each of the processes developed thus far transform into time and resource gaps for submitters. These biomarker qualification process gaps are not easily bridged, and are major hurdles in the completion of qualification processes.

Divergent development of biomarker qualification processes in different regulatory agencies is an additional hurdle, because these divergent processes also result in a divergent list of qualified biomarkers. This is an unacceptable outcome, which has the potential to impact the harmonization of regulatory review for drug approvals. These divergent qualification processes need to be harmonized soon, perhaps with an extension of the ICH E16 document. Ultimately, an independent international biomarker qualification process will be needed to support a harmonized qualified biomarker infrastructure for drug development around the world.

References

[1] US FDA. Guidance for Industry – Pharmacogenomic Data Submissions. www.fda.gov/downloads/ RegulatoryInformation/Guidances/UCM126957.pdf; 2005. Accessed June 10, 2013.

[2] US FDA. Critical Path Opportunities List. www.fda.gov/downloads/scienceresearch/specialtopics/ CriticalPathinitiative/CriticalPathOpportunitiesreports/UCM077258.pdf; 2006. Accessed June 10, 2013.

[3] Altar CA, Amakye D, Bounos D, Bloom J, Clack G, Dean R, et al. A Prototypical Process for Creating Evidentiary Standards for Biomarkers and Diagnostics. Clin Pharmacol Ther 2008;83(2):368–71.

[4] Institute of Medicine of the National Academy of Sciences (US). Consensus Report. Evaluation of Biomarkers and Surrogate Endpoints in Chronic Disease 2010.

[5] Woodcock J, Importance of genomic biomarker validation in the context of pharmacogenomic initiatives at the FDA. Pharmacogenomics in Drug Development and Regulatory Decision Making – Workshop 3: Three Years of Promise, Proposals, and Progress on Optimizing the Benefit/Risk of Medicines. Bethesda, MD: Co-sponsored by DIA, FDA, PWG, PhRMA & BIO, 4/11–13/2005; 2005.

[6] Goodsaid FM, Frueh F. Chapter 9. Regulatory Guidance and Validation of Toxicologic Biomarkers. In: DeCaprio AP, editor. Toxicologic Biomarkers. New York: Taylor & Francis Group; 2006. p. 187–200.

[7] Goodsaid FM, Frueh F. Process Map Proposal for the Validation of Genomic Biomarkers. Pharmacogenomics 2006;7(5):773–82.

[8] US FDA. Guidance for Industry. Qualification Process for Drug Development Tools, http://www. fda.gov/downloads/Drugs/GuidanceComplianceRegulatoryInformation/Guidances/UCM230597. pdf; 2010. Accessed June 10, 2013.

[9] Goodsaid FM, Frueh FW, Mattes W. Strategic Paths for Biomarker Qualification. Toxicology 2008; 245:219–23.

[10] FNIH Biomarkers Consortium, www.biomarkersconsortium.org. Accessed June 10, 2013.

[11] Woosley RL, Myers RT, Goodsaid FM. The Critical Path Institute's approach to precompetitive sharing and advancing regulatory science. Clin Pharmacol Ther 2010;87:530–3.

[12] Dieterle F, Sistare F, Goodsaid F, Papaluca M, Ozer JS, Webb CP, et al. Renal biomarker qualification submission: a dialog between the FDA-EMEA and predictive safety testing consortium. Nat Biotechnol 2010;28:455–62.

[13] US FDA. Review Submission of the Qualification of Seven Biomarkers of Drug-Induced Nephrotoxicity in rats, http://www.fda.gov/downloads/Drugs/DevelopmentApprovalProcess/ DrugDevelopmentToolsQualificationProgram/UCM285031.pdf; 2008. Accessed June 10, 2013.

[14] US FDA. FDA Biomarker Qualification Process, http://www.fda.gov/Drugs/DevelopmentApproval Process/DrugDevelopmentToolsQualificationProgram/ucm284621.htm; 2011. Accessed June 10, 2013.

[15] EMA. EMA Biomarker Qualification Process, http://www.ema.europa.eu/docs/en_GB/document_ library/Regulatory_and_procedural_guideline/2009/10/WC500004201.pdf; 2009. Accessed June 10, 2013.

[16] Romero K, de Mars M, Frank D, Anthony M, Neville J, Kirby L, et al. The Coalition Against Major Diseases: Developing Tools for an Integrated Drug Development Process for Alzheimer's and Parkinsosn's Diseases. Clin Pharm Therapeutics 2009;86(4):365–7.

[17] CAMD. Coalition Against Major Diseases. http://c-path.org/CAMDPipeline.cfm; 2008. Accessed June 10, 2013.

[18] Isaac M, Vamvakas S, Abadie E, Jonsson B, Gispen C, Pani L. Qualification opinion of novel methodologies in the predementia stage of Alzheimer's disease: cerebro-spinal-fluid related bio-markers for drugs affecting amyloid burden – regulatory considerations by European Medicines Agency focusing on improving benefit/risk in regulatory trials. Eur Neuropsychopharmacol 2011; 21(11):781–8.

[19] EMA. EMA Qualification for Alzheimer Biomarkers, http://www.ema.europa.eu/docs/en_GB/document_library/Regulatory_and_procedural_guideline/2012/04/WC500125018.pdf; 2012. Accessed June 10, 2013.

[20] ICH. Biomarkers Related to Drug or Biotechnology Product Development: Context, Structure and Format of Qualification Submissions. http://www.ich.org/fileadmin/Public_Web_Site/ICH_Products/Guidelines/Efficacy/E16/Step4/E16_Step_4.pdf; 2010. Accessed June 10, 2013.

[21] FDA. Guidance for Industry. E16 Biomarkers Related to Drug or Biotechnology Product Development: Context, Structure, and Format of Qualification Submissions, http://www.fda.gov/downloads/Drugs/GuidanceComplianceRegulatoryInformation/Guidances/UCM267449.pdf; 2011. Accessed June 10, 2013.

[22] http://ihcp.jrc.ec.europa.eu/our_labs/euriecvam. Accessed June 10, 2013.

3

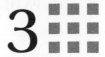

Regulatory Experience of Biomarker Qualification in the EMA

Spiros Vamvakas

HEAD OF SCIENTIFIC ADVICE, EUROPEAN MEDICINES AGENCY, LONDON, UK

The EMEA qualification process launched in 2009 is a new, voluntary, scientific pathway leading to either a Committee for Human Medicinal Products (CHMP) opinion or a Scientific Advice on innovative methods or drug development tools. These two outcomes are distinguished as:

- CHMP Qualification Advice on future protocols and methods for further method development towards qualification, based on the evaluation of the scientific rationale and on preliminary data submitted.
- CHMP Qualification Opinion on the acceptability of a specific use of the proposed method; e.g., use of a novel methodology or an imaging method in a research and development (R&D) context (non-clinical or clinical studies), based on the assessment of submitted data.

The qualification process addresses the implementation of innovative drug development methods and tools. It focuses on the use of novel methodologies developed by consortia, networks, public/private partnerships, learned societies and the pharmaceutical industry for a specific intended use in pharmaceuticals research and development. New development methods include, for example, pharmacogenomics, proteomics, patient and provider reported outcome scales, and imaging procedures such as MRI and PET; such methods may be used as inclusion criteria in clinical trials or to monitor disease progression. The qualification procedure may be linked to the development of one or more specific products. The Applicant can submit an application for a Qualification Advice on how to develop a new method, or if they are of the view that they have already completed the development required for the qualification, they can opt to directly submit an application for a Qualification Opinion. If the Agency agrees the data support qualification, a Qualification Opinion is issued (see below). If the Agency is of the view that further studies are required, the procedure is converted into a Qualification Advice and the Applicant receives a response on what additional studies are needed.

It should be noted that the <u>existing</u> Scientific Advice/Protocol Assistance procedure is prospective advice related to specific products, indications, or technology within a development program. The existing Scientific Advice/Protocol Assistance procedure is not affected by the new qualification procedure.

The Path from Biomarker Discovery to Regulatory Qualification. http://dx.doi.org/10.1016/B978-0-12-391496-5.00003-X

The primary evaluation for qualification is carried out by a team appointed in the Scientific Advice Working Party (SAWP) of the CHMP. This specialized team ('Qualification Team'), which is led by a Coordinator who is a CHMP and/or SAWP member, oversees the preparatory assessment of data and protocols and ensures that efficient use is made of the resources available in the EMEA experts' network. The procedure to provide this broad scientific advice is based on the existing Scientific Advice procedure but is adapted to host the activity of the Qualification Team and to incorporate international collaboration. During the evaluation there is at least one face-to-face meeting between the Applicant and the Qualification Team.

In the case of a Qualification opinion, a public consultation step is additionally implemented to gather the views of the scientific community prior to a final Qualification Opinion. The public consultation of the scientific community will ensure that CHMP/SAWP shares information and is open to broad-based scientific scrutiny and discussion. The timing of the public consultation is determined in agreement with the Applicant, who then also has the opportunity to remove any confidential information from the document to be published.

It is up to the Applicant to contact agencies other than the EMEA before the start of the procedure. While there was extensive preparatory informal work between the FDA (Food and Drugs Administration) and EMA before the launching of the formal EMA procedure, there is no formal parallel Qualification Advice with any other agency. There is, however, the confidentiality agreement between the FDA/PMDA and the EMA which makes it possible to have a qualification proceeding in parallel and at the same time in more than one agency, offering the Applicant the opportunity for input from more than one agency. However, if the Applicant wishes to include more than one agency in the qualification process, appropriate arrangements should be established before the start of the procedure. While an Applicant can certainly request that a specific procedure is handled by the EMA only, Applicants are encouraged to apply in parallel to the EMEA and FDA. The agencies then communicate the assessment and meet with the Applicant together. This maximizes the chance for scientific consensus. Indeed, for the purpose of scientific consensus the FDA and EMA have set up quarterly teleconferences during which the experts informally discuss ongoing qualification procedures which have not been submitted to the Agencies as formal parallel procedures.

In conclusion, the 'Qualification of Novel Methodologies' through the SAWP of the CHMP is a formal procedure resulting either in a Qualification Advice or a Qualification Opinion.

Other Informal Interactions with the EMA

Informal briefing meetings with the Pharmacogenomics Working Party and other experts on development of novel biomarkers are still taking place (before the procedure of qualification of novel methodologies) and are encouraged in an early stage of development. Briefing meetings normally occur once on each specific approach and do not result in a document expressing the CHMP opinion on the issues discussed. The sponsor is recommended to seek the new qualification procedure after the briefing meeting. Briefing meetings should not occur during the qualification procedure. Meetings with the Innovation Task Force are not affected by the new procedure(s).

Examples of Qualification Opinions

In the three years since EMA has launched the Procedure, the agency has engaged in 24 Qualification Advices (finalized and ongoing) and six Qualification Opinions (five published and one in preparation at the time this chapter was being written). Examples of the published Qualification Opinions can be found below.

1. Qualification Opinion of Low Hippocampal Volume (atrophy) by MRI for Use in Clinical Trials for Regulatory Purposes – in the Predementia Stage of Alzheimer's Disease

The present opinion addresses the question of whether the use of baseline measurement of low hippocampal volume (atrophy) by MRI is qualified in selecting (i.e., to categorize) subjects for trials in early Alzheimer's disease (AD) as having a high probability of being in the prodromal stage of the disease as defined by the Dubois Criteria (2007).

CHMP Discussion

The relative value of this biomarker compared to other potential biomarkers (e.g., cerebral spinal fluid [CSF] analytes), or compared to other characteristics associated with the rate of conversion to AD (e.g., age and cognitive tests) is still not fully established. The *de novo* analyses performed by the Sponsor on the Alzheimer's Disease Neuroimaging Initiative (ADNI) dataset show a statistically significant association of MRI hippocampal volume with conversion to AD. The association appears strong enough to accept its qualification for the intended purpose. It would have been desirable to be able to assess the independent value of this MRI biomarker in terms of its predictive value as a single dichotomized marker (low vs. normal volume), assessing it independently of the value of other determinants of conversion such as age and cognitive tests (ADAS-cog) which have been considered simultaneously in the prognostic model. However, this is difficult with the data currently available. To facilitate the design of the intended 'enriched' clinical trials, it would have been useful to characterize the conversion free survival functions according to the studied MRI biomarker, describing the probability of conversion for different time points for those with MRI low hippocampal volume and those with normal MRI images but, again, this is difficult with the available datasets.

CHMP Qualification Opinion

Low hippocampal volume, as measured by MRI and considered as a dichotomized variable (low volume or not), might be considered a marker of progression to dementia in subjects with cognitive deficit compatible with predementia stage of AD (Dubois, 2007). For the purposes of enriching a clinical trial population. As such, low hippocampal volume may facilitate enriched clinical trials aimed at studying drugs which potentially slow the progress/conversion to AD-dementia of the included subjects. However, neither the actual value of low hippocampal volume to accurately predict rate of such progression to dementia in the referred subjects nor the relative value of other biomarkers have been reported.

Currently envisioned in the current opinion is that subjects might be included in future studies based on clinical criteria and the low hippocampal volume biomarker (if positive). The CHMP has given a previous positive opinion in the use of cerebrospinal fluid-related biomarkers in the predementia stage of AD for drugs affecting amyloid burden. This may lead first to a heterogeneous population and, moreover, it will not be possible to explore the relationship among them. The concurrent assessment of other qualified biomarkers in predementia AD would be highly desirable and of great value. Collection, handling and measurements of low hippocampal volume, as measured by MRI, should be performed according to Good Clinical Practice and to the specific highest international standards for these measurements. Low hippocampal volume, as measured by MRI, is not qualified as a diagnostic tool or outcome or longitudinal measure.

2. Qualification Opinion of Novel Methodologies in the Predementia Stage of AD: Cerebrospinal Fluid-Related Biomarkers for Drugs Affecting Amyloid Burden

The present opinion addresses the question of whether the use of two CSF-related biomarkers ($A\beta$1–42 and total tau 1) are qualified in selecting (i.e., to categorize) subjects for trials in early AD as having a high probability of being in the prodromal stage of the disease as defined by the Dubois Criteria (2007).

CHMP Qualification Opinion

In patients with Mild Cognitive Impairment (MCI), a positive CSF biomarker signature based on a low $A\beta$1–42 and a high T-tau can help predict evolution to AD-dementia type. The positive predictive value (PPV) is at least 60%. Given the relatively high sensitivity and moderate specificity, the CSF biomarker signature based on a low $A\beta$1–42 and a high T-tau is useful for the enrichment of clinical trial populations. ELISA methods to measure this CSF biomarker signature are commercially available, but the measurement process is complex. Reliable results require the standardization of all steps, from liquor collection and the type of vials used in sampling to the last working procedure in the circuit. Accordingly, international guidelines have been produced to assure inter-site concordance; these guidelines must be enforced. The CSF biomarker signature based on a low $A\beta$1–42 and a high T-tau is qualified to identify MCI patients who most nearly equate to the prodromal stage of AD (Dubois et al., 2007) and who are at risk to evolve into AD-dementia. Collection, handling and measurements of all CSF samples should be performed according to Good Laboratory Practice and to the specific international standards for these measurements.

3. Qualification Opinion of Alzheimer's Disease Novel Methodologies/ Biomarkers for PET Amyloid Imaging (Positive/Negative) for Use in Enrichment Strategies for Predementia AD Clinical Trials

In follow-up to the positive Qualification Opinion on the use of cerebrospinal fluid (CSF) biomarkers in predementia AD adopted on 14-Apr-2011 (EMA/CHMP/SAWP/102001/2011) the Applicant requested Qualification opinion of Alzheimer's disease novel methodologies/biomarkers for PET amyloid imaging (positive/negative) as a biomarker for enrichment for use in predementia AD clinical trials and to expand the Qualification opinion of Alzheimer's disease novel methodologies/biomarkers for PET amyloid imaging (positive/negative) as a biomarker for enrichment for use in predementia AD clinical trials.

CHMP Qualification Opinion on PET Biomarker Signature

Amyloid-related positive/negative PET signal is considered qualified to identify patients with clinical diagnosis of predementia AD who are at increased risk of having an underlying AD neuropathology, for the purposes of enriching a clinical trial population. However, neither the actual value of PET (+) or (−) to accurately predict rate of such progression to dementia in the referred subjects, nor the relative value of other biomarkers have been reported. Thus, we recommended to follow up these patients until clinical diagnosis of Mild AD is made. Collection, handling and measurements of all PET signals should be performed according to Good Clinical Practice and to the specific highest international standards for these measurements. The concurrent assessment of recently qualified biomarkers in the predementia stage of AD would be highly desirable and of great value. Amyloid-related positive/negative PET is not qualified as a diagnostic tool or outcome or longitudinal measure.

4.   Qualification Opinion ILSI/HESI Submission of Novel Renal Biomarkers for Toxicity

The HESI study evaluated four novel urinary biomarkers (BMs) of nephrotoxicity, i.e., alpha-glutathioneS-transferase (α-GST), μ-glutathione S-transferase (μ-GST), renal papillary antigen-1 (RPA-1) and clusterin, and compared their performance against the more traditional measurements for diagnosing nephrotoxicity. The data presented in this report were all generated in single and repeated dose studies conducted in male rats of two strains (Sprague-Dawley and Wistar) that are commonly used in preclinical toxicity studies. The information obtained from these studies demonstrates the potential utility of these BMs for use in rodent studies conducted to evaluate the potential target organ toxicity of compounds as part of the preclinical safety assessment of candidate medicines.

CHMP Qualification Opinion

Clusterin was previously qualified by the FDA and the European Medicines agency after review of the PSTC submission (published report: http://www.emea.europa.eu/pdfs/human/sciadvice/67971908en.pdf):

> *'The urinary kidney BMs (Kim-1, Albumin, Total Protein, β2-Microglobulin, Urinary Clusterin, Urinary Trefoil Factor 3 and Urinary Cystatin C) are considered acceptable in the context of non-clinical drug development for the detection of acute drug-induced nephrotoxicity, either tubular or glomerular with associated tubular involvement. They provide additional and complementary information to Blood*

Urea Nitrogen (BUN) and Serum Creatinine to correlate with histo-pathological alterations considered to be the gold standard. Additional data on the correlation between the BMs and the evolution and reversibility, of acute kidney injury are needed. Also, further knowledge on species-specificity is required.'

The findings of the current HESI submission increase the level of evidence supporting the use of Urinary Clusterin. Urinary Clusterin is a biomarker that may be used by Applicants to detect acute drug-induced renal tubule alterations, particularly when regeneration is present, in male rats and can be included along with traditional clinical chemistry markers and histopathology in GLP toxicology studies which are used to support renal safety in clinical trials. In addition, the HESI data indicate that urinary RPA-1 is a biomarker that may be used to detect acute drug-induced renal tubular alterations, particularly in the collecting duct, in male rats, and can be included along with traditional clinical chemistry markers and histopathology in GLP toxicology studies which are used to support renal safety in clinical trials. The Qualification Team acknowledges that the HESI data may support the use of urinary α-GST in detecting proximal tubule injury in male rats. However the opposing effects of proximal and collecting duct injury on α-GST levels raise uncertainty about the usefulness of this biomarker for detecting mild early renal injury. Therefore before α-GST is qualified in this context further studies will be needed to evaluate the mechanistic basis and usefulness of this BM.

CHMP Recommendations towards Future Qualification Experiments

METHODOLOGICAL CONSIDERATIONS

- Replication of evidence: the conclusions drawn can be made more robust if replicated evidence is available from another, similar series of experiments.
- Biomarker normalization: For all urinary markers, analyte concentrations for all animals were first normalized by dividing by the corresponding urine creatinine concentration. All individual animal marker values (normalized to creatinine in the case of urinary markers) were divided by the mean of the values in the concurrent control (i.e., vehicle-dosed) animals. Thus, all marker values were expressed as a fold-change versus the time-matched control group mean. Urine creatinine normalization of BMs values is a standard practice and is considered acceptable. However normalization of the urinary BMs by the mean of the values in the concurrent control is not recommended. It is acknowledged that this is done to minimize the impact of inter-study variability in the BMs performance. However, the BMs should be normalized to the individual baseline BMs values. Since urine baseline data was not collected in this experiment it is recommended to conduct this normalization in future studies. The Applicant argues that intra-animal variability is greater than inter-animal, suggesting that baseline data may be of limited value with respect to variance reduction. However both Applicant and QT agree that collection of baseline data in future studies will be beneficial.

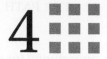

4

Regulatory Experience at the FDA, EMA, and PMDA
Regulatory Experience at the PMDA

Akihiro Ishiguro, Yasuto Otsubo, Yoshiaki Uyama

*PMDA OMICS PROJECT (POP), PHARMACEUTICALS AND MEDICAL
DEVICES AGENCY, TOKYO, JAPAN*

Pharmacogenomics (PGx) and biomarkers have gradually been recognized as useful tools for use throughout the life cycle of a drug or device, from development through post-approval activities. In September 2005, the Japanese Pharmaceuticals and Medical Devices Agency (PMDA) established the PGx Discussion Group (PDG) to appropriately manage PGx issues in Japan's regulatory process. The PDG only covered PGx issues, but recently, interest in other 'omics' areas, such as proteomics, metabonomics and metabolomics have rapidly increased. Therefore, in April 2009, the PDG was re-organized as the PMDA Omics Project (POP), which covers not only PGx but also proteomics, metabonomics, metabolomics and related issues.

The mission of POP is summarized in Table 4.1.

At the same time as POP was established, PMDA also created a new and formal scientific consultation process focusing on PGx/biomarkers. Since then, POP has been responsible for this formal consultation. The outline for the formal consultation process for PGx/biomarkers, such as the purpose and timeline of the consultation, and the qualification process for a biomarker, is described in Chapter 19. POP currently consists of 27 members from various offices in PMDA, such as the Office of Regulatory Science, the Office of New Drug I-V, the Office of Cellular and Tissue-based Products, the Office of Vaccines and Blood Products, the Office of Medical Devices, the Office of Safety, the Office of Compliance and the Office of Review Management, to cover broader topics relating to omics (as of April 2013). To achieve its mission, beyond the formal scientific consultation, POP conducts informal discussion meetings with industry or academia as well as internal meetings on a regular basis. The informal discussion meetings (POP meetings) provide an

Table 4.1 Mission of POP

- Share data, information, and knowledge relating to omics
- Discuss regulatory issues related to omics
- Maintain decision consistency among reviewers and offices within PMDA
- Evaluate omics data that are not directly related to individual drug/diagnostic device developments

The Path from Biomarker Discovery to Regulatory Qualification. http://dx.doi.org/10.1016/B978-0-12-391496-5.00004-1

opportunity for experts from academia and industry to communicate with PMDA, without constraint, regarding the latest scientific data and information. Such communications are also important for PMDA to remain up-to-date with the latest science and research in the fields of PGx and biomarkers. Through these actions, POP plays an active role in promoting PGx- and biomarker-based drug and device development.

Recently, PMDA has reviewed numerous new drug applications (NDAs) and conducted scientific consultations regarding clinical development in PGx and biomarkers. Examples of drug developments in these fields in Japan are the clinical trials of bapineuzumab in patients with Alzheimer's disease who carry ApoE4, and the clinical trials of mogamulizumab in patients with C-C chemokine receptor type 4-positive adult T cell leukemia-lymphoma [1,2]. Moreover, the use of PGx and biomarkers in the post-approval stage has increased annually in Japan. According to our study, 10–15 % of new drug labels (prescribing information) in Japan include information regarding PGx/biomarkers, such as polymorphisms of the genes coding for drug metabolizing enzymes and the target molecule of a drug [3,4]. In addition to the labels of recently approved new drugs, many labels of old drugs have also been revised to include newly available scientific information derived from PGx and biomarker studies. For example, in 2008, the label of irinotecan was revised to include the information about an increased risk of serious neutropenia in patients who are homozygous for *UGT1A1*6* or **28*, or heterozygously carrying a combination of both of *UGT1A1*6* and **28* [5]. The Japanese regulatory body (Ministry of Health, Labor and Welfare, and PMDA) had encouraged companies to develop a genetic test device for the UGT1A1 polymorphism. This resulted in the approval of an *in vitro* companion *in vitro* diagnostics device (IVD), the INVADER® UGT1A1 assay, for genotyping of *UGT1A1*6* and **28* at the same time as the label was updated [6]. More recently, the label of carbamazepine was revised to include the information about the association between serious cutaneous adverse drug reactions like Stevens-Johnson Syndrome, and the genetic polymorphism of the human leukocytic antigen, *HLA-A*3103*, based on the Japanese population data reported by Ozeki et al. [7,8].

As described above, although PGx/biomarker data submission to PMDA has been popularized, challenges remain for further implementation of PGx/biomarker utility in Japan. For example, in our recent studies, companion IVDs has not been approved for approximately half of the biomarkers identified in the labels of new drugs in Japan [3], and many differences in the contexts (contents and descriptions) of PGx/biomarker information have been identified in Japanese and US drug labels [9]. PMDA has been working to promote the co-development of drugs and companion IVDs, and the accumulation of PGx/biomarker data in clinical trials. However, more international collaborations between PMDA and other international organizations such as regulatory agencies, industry, and academia are necessary to promote PGx- and biomarker-based drug and device development. For example, in clinical trials, samples for genetic tests should be collected to the extent possible to enable better assessment of the data. Currently, however, the collection rate of DNA samples is not high in global clinical trials, possibly due to difference in regulatory requirements and the reviews by ethics committees in each country [10]. In such cases, an international guideline would facilitate the process of sampling and accumulating PGx/biomarker evidence in a standardized manner acceptable to all regions. In the era of globalization, a regulatory agency cannot achieve its mission to protect and promote public health without international collaborations, and the roles of regulatory agencies in these collaborations have become more important. Therefore, further collaboration among regulatory agencies should be encouraged.

In recent years, PMDA has also reinforced its ability to conduct in-house research activities in regulatory science [11]. Accumulated research outcomes will be useful to facilitate a scientific discussion among regulatory agencies, industry and academia. These outcomes will also assist in the establishment of more international standards or guidelines to implement the use of PGx/biomarker data in drug and device developments, as well as in clinical practice. PMDA will continue to promote innovative scientific tools that allow better drugs and devices to become available to patients.

Acknowledgment

The views expressed in this chapter are those of the authors and do not necessarily reflect the official views of the Pharmaceuticals and Medical Devices Agency.

References

[1] Clinical Trials.gov, the US National Institutes of Health. Bapineuzumab in patients with mild to moderate Alzheimer's disease (ApoE4 Carrier) http://www.clinicaltrials.gov/ct2/show/NCT00575055?term=AAB-001&phase=2&rank=5 (accessed on June 14th, 2013).

[2] Clinical Trials.gov, the US National Institutes of Health. Multicenter, randomized, open-label, parallel-group study to compare mLSG15 + KW-0761 to mLSG15 http://www.clinicaltrials.gov/ct2/show/NCT01173887?term=kw0761&rank=1 (accessed on June 14th, 2013).

[3] Kadowaki K, Ishiguro A, Takamatsu S, Saito Y, Uyama Y. Analytical consideration on pharmacogenomics information in the package inserts of drugs and availability of genetic tests in Japan. Regulatory Sci Med Products 2012;2:83–91.

[4] Ishiguro A, Toyoshima S, Uyama Y. Current Japanese regulatory situations of pharmacogenomics in drug administration. Exp Rev Clin Pharmacol 2008;1:505–14.

[5] Database for drug label information (in Japanese), Pharmaceuticals and Medical Devices Agency, Notification of instruction to revise label of irinotecan http://www.info.pmda.go.jp/kaiteip/20080616B/01.pdf (accessed on June 14th, 2013).

[6] Pharmaceuticals and Medical Devices Safety Information No.235, Ministry of Health Labour and Welfare, Overview of Pharmacogenomics http://www.pmda.go.jp/english/service/pdf/precautions/PMDSI-235.pdf (accessed on June 14th, 2013).

[7] Pharmaceuticals and Medical Devices Safety Information No.285, Ministry of Health Labour and Welfare. Carbamazepine-induced serious drug eruption and genetic polymorphism http://www.pmda.go.jp/english/service/pdf/precautions/PMDSI-285.pdf (accessed on June 14th, 2013).

[8] Ozeki T, Mushiroda T, Yowang A, Takahashi A, Kubo M, Shirakata Y, et al. Genome-wide association study identifies *HLA-A*3101* allele as a genetic risk factor for carbamazepine-induced cutaneous adverse drug reactions in Japanese population. Hum Mol Genet 2011;20:1034–41.

[9] Otsubo Y, Asahina Y, Noguchi A, Sato Y, Ando Y, Uyama Y. Similarities and differences between US and Japan as to pharmacogenomic biomarker information in drug lables. Drug Metab Pharmacokinet 2012;27:142–9.

[10] Warner AW. Challenges in obtaining adequate genetic sample sets in clinical trials: the perspective of the industry pharmacogenomics working group. Clin Pharmacol Ther 2011;89:529–36.

[11] Asahina Y, Tanaka A, Uyama Y, Kuramochi K, Maruyama H. The roles of regulatory science research in drug development at the Pharmaceuticals and Medical Devices Agency of Japan. Therapeutic Innovation and Regulatory Science 2013;47:19–22.

Biomarker Development and Qualification in the Pharmaceutical Industry

5

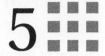

The Impact of Changing Context of Use on Weight of Evidence for Qualification of Biomarkers: A Case Study in Ischemic Stroke

Stephen A. Williams

SOMATOLOGIC INC., BOULDER, CO, USA

My favorite catchphrase about biomarkers is 'fitness for purpose', which is included in most people's definitions of qualification. My second favorite is 'reasonably likely' which isn't often included in definitions, but is in the Federal Code of Regulations about the predictions from surrogate endpoints in accelerated approval and also in the Pharmaceutical Research Manufactures Association (PhRMA) position paper on proof of concept. My third favorite is 'truth standard'. I like these mental shortcuts because they include key (albeit hidden) principles of good practice (in bold below and in the case study) which are adaptable to many different circumstances. The 'fitness' principle is that the **nature of the evidence** acquired must support the purpose, and 'purpose' requires a predefined **intended use and context of use**. The 'reasonably likely' principle is a combination of 'reasonably' which requires an assessment of the **weight of evidence** one might require for acceptance in the intended use (a risk/benefit assessment) and 'likely' which is a **probability** assessment about what outcomes are most likely and whether that required weight of evidence has been met. The **'truth standard'** principle asks what measure of truth we are using today to capture the effect that we are asking the biomarker to represent, and how good it is. If the truth standard is poor, a perfect biomarker will be poorly correlated with it, and will appear to be poor as well. Unfortunately, while all those phrases beautifully capture the concealed principles, their very concealment, the absence of a rigorous discipline around qualification, and their subjectivity, means that they can be trumped unintentionally or intentionally by human factors and changing circumstances. These human factors are discussed in the story shown below, which has been anonymized to protect the innocent.

The biomarker in this story is diffusion-weighted MRI (magnetic resonance imaging); specifically the growth of the affected edematous area in the brain during the first 24–48h after an ischemic stroke in humans. While the therapeutic area of stroke is an area of high medical need, the exploratory clinical development path was, and still is, a nightmare for two reasons. The first reason is that the Food and Drugs Administration (FDA)-accepted clinical or neurological outcomes assessments are variable, subjective and require several months of follow-up. In exploratory development, where most drugs fail, the cost to reach a decision is high. Statistically, the success rate in Phase II studies in stroke is pretty dreadful, so the cost per success can reach uneconomic levels for a commercial organization. The second reason is that the clinical outcome in stroke depends on the size of the stroke (which *can* be improved by a drug) and the site of the stroke in the brain (which *cannot* be changed by a drug). As a **truth standard** for pharmacological benefit, the clinical outcome measures are therefore flawed: a small stroke in your motor cortex would have a profound effect on your neurological score, whereas a large one in your frontal cortex could just cause you to make socially inappropriate remarks. This means that the pharmacological signal-to-noise ratio is inevitably poor, even for an effective drug. We were therefore interested in MRI for the **intended use** of detecting the key element of our drug's pharmacologic mechanism (reduction in growth of the edema) and reducing the cost of a likely no-go decision in exploratory development. The **context of use** at the time was that the portfolio in the company as a whole was quite rich and healthy, and there was considerable support for the concept of 'proof of non-viability' using biomarkers and novel technologies. The pharmacology to which the technology would be applied depended on the theory of preventing the spread of the 'cytotoxic edema' around a stroke after the initial ischemic insult.

Considering the **nature of evidence** to demonstrate fitness for this purpose, the key requirement would be that the technology should be capable of detecting the spread of cytotoxic edema. We determined that this evidence was available. Diffusion MRI is inherently designed to measure edema and in preclinical experiments correlated with the areas of the brain which were histopathologically edematous. We had also already run a natural history study using diffusion MRI in ~20 humans in untreated stroke, which showed that we could measure a doubling in size of the edematous area in humans in the first 48 hours after the ischemic insult. As a **truth standard** for the amount of edema, MRI therefore looked pretty good. We did not know from MRI whether this edema was indeed mediated by cytotoxicity, but this was not a risk in making a correct no-go decision because if it wasn't cytotoxic then the pharmacology of the drug wouldn't work anyway! We determined that we did not need to demonstrate a linkage to clinical outcomes with MRI because we were using it simply to detect the presence or absence of the relevant pharmacological mechanistic effect, not using it to claim that this effect (if present) would lead to a clinical benefit. It was also clear that the clinical **truth standard** is poor, so that even if MRI had been a perfect outcomes measure, the correlation between it and the existing clinical scores could only be modest at best. Note how the utility of this biomarker is asymmetric: it has a higher degree of accuracy in predicting a correct 'no-go' decision (when the intended pharmacology is absent), but it is weaker in predicting a correct 'go' decision (when the pharmacology is present but we don't know whether it leads to a real benefit).

Regarding the **weight of evidence** that would make it 'reasonably likely' that the biomarker is qualified, we must consider the consequences of each true and false decision outcome. A true positive is a neutral result – the probability of clinical success is only slightly increased because we don't know whether a biomarker positive predicts improved outcome. This might have a benefit of enabling an increase in the investment in Phase IIb, but conversely we need to catch up just to stand still because we've already delayed the program by inserting a critical path MRI study that turned out not to be necessary. A true negative result is valuable: cost-effectively terminating the program early, saving fully absorbed costs of many millions of dollars and similar opportunity costs. A false positive is fairly neutral (aside from the study costs of the MRI study), as it would lead to the same futile Phase II study that would have been done without the MRI program. A false negative would lead to an inappropriate termination decision, which is harmful with the lost benefits to patients and the lost revenues to the company, but given the rich portfolio of 'replacement' programs is not a great threat to the future of the company. Considering what is the most **likely** outcome – when the history of clinical development is littered with many failed compounds in stroke – a negative decision is statistically the most **probable**.

Given that the value (of success) or harm (of failure) of the biomarker for this purpose is mostly driven by the negative results, and that such negative results are most **probable**, there should be a **high weight of evidence** that the test should correctly identify a drug's failure to reduce cytotoxic edema (it should have a high negative predictive value – NPV). Given that true or false positive results are of low harm and low value, there should be a **low weight of evidence** that the test should predict clinical outcome (it doesn't need a high positive predictive value – PPV). In conclusion, retrospectively applying this discipline, it does seem **reasonably likely** that diffusion MRI in humans was more than adequately qualified for the **intended use** of making a proof of non-viability decision for a pharmacology related to cytotoxic edema.

In fact, the Phase IIa study was run using diffusion-weighted MRI in about 40 subjects per group (placebo vs. active), with special care to standardize the measurement and image analyses, and it was clearly negative. There was not a trace of a difference: the placebo and drug groups' growth of edema profiles on MRI were superimposable, and, gratifyingly, both were within a few percent of the prior natural history study. This showed that the technology had performed consistently across studies. The governance body agreed that this was a clear no-go decision and the program was terminated.

Except that it wasn't.

Fast forward a year or so and the **context of use** had changed. The organization could see a gap in products in development, and a problem with patent expirations. It needed to fill the gap. The drug development team in neurodegeneration had no products in development. A team of committed scientists and doctors still desperately wanted to help patients. In other words, because of the change in **context,** what was considered **'reasonable'** had changed. The **weight of evidence** that one might need to advance a drug was justifiably lower and the **weight of evidence** for a termination decision higher. Of course this is the rationalization of hindsight – at the time everyone appeared to be acting on intuition.

In the new context, the study decision was re-evaluated by a new team. The diffusion MRI technique was now viewed as inadequate because it did not (in the literature) clearly relate to clinical outcome and was not viewed by FDA as an acceptable endpoint. The failure here was that the disciplined arguments made above – that linkage to outcome was not necessary for a characterization of pharmacology, and that it was not even likely to be good given the poor clinical **truth standard** – were not written down in anticipation of this argument. There was no explicit record that this was supposed to be a clinical pharmacology proof of non-viability experiment. When these arguments above were used to counter the team's new critique of MRI at the time, the opinions were inevitably discounted by a conflict of interests: the leadership of the technology group, of course, would be reluctant to admit that it was wrong and MRI didn't work after all. The methods of rationalizing and describing asymmetric biomarker predictions (that for this purpose the NPV was more important than PPV) had not yet been developed as described above. The governance body had changed (I was no longer on it!). We had even received a letter from the FDA during the MRI study saying that they viewed MRI as an unvalidated surrogate endpoint, requesting that we change the primary analysis of the study to be based on clinical outcomes. We had declined this at the time because it was a Phase IIa mechanistic pharmacology study. Now that the weight of evidence required for a termination decision had increased, it was easy to say that MRI was no longer '**reasonably likely**' to be qualified.

Similarly, with the **weight of evidence** for a 'go' decision substantially reduced by operational needs, a new statistical analysis of the outcomes data collected in the MRI study was commissioned. The statistical analysis predefined in the protocol showed no significant difference in outcomes, but it was under-powered for an outcomes study at only 40 patients per group. Initially, there wasn't a numerical difference between placebo and drug in the key neurological outcome measure (dichotomized NIH stroke scale – DNIHSS) at the final visit. However, over a period of many months, a number of different analyses were done. The team cleverly discovered that although the mild and moderate strokes were well matched in the placebo and drug group before treatment, by random chance the serious ones with scores above 20 were more serious in the drug group. So a group-wide statistical adjustment was made for seriousness at baseline and, as a result, the drug treated group did better than placebo and this reached statistical significance. This was sufficient for a 'go' decision.

At the time, I did not see it so benignly – after all I was defending my personal interests as a purveyor of technology which could improve productivity in drug development. But now I can understand the substantial shift that had taken place in decision-making when the organization was desperate for more products. I had not grasped that the **weight of evidence** for 'go' and 'no-go' decisions had flipped from high/low when the program started to low/high later. My actions included obtaining opinions from a different 'rival' group of statisticians within the company, not involved with this project, who told me that the statistical adjustment was inappropriately done, and the many post-hoc analyses weren't corrected for multiple comparisons. These arguments fell on deaf ears. What I failed to realize is that the **context of use** had changed so substantially.

The program was resurrected and a decision-making clinical outcomes trial in stroke was run. It was terminated due to futility three years later.

It is tempting to say that we had created the worst economic scenario for the company: the development team (including me) had more than doubled the cost of a 'no-go' decision by making the organization pay for two sequential futile studies (when only one should have done the trick). However, on a portfolio level this is not necessarily true. Did the change in context, requiring a lower weight of evidence for 'go' decisions and a higher weight of evidence for 'no-go' decisions', when applied across the portfolio, lead to a resurrection or advancement of other compounds which did make it? Or conversely, did it lead to even more futile expense!? To answer that would require a portfolio analysis which I have not done.

This case study enabled me to learn several important lessons. The first is that biomarker qualification should become a rigorous discipline which requires explicit definitions of the **intended use and context, the nature of evidence, the weight of evidence and the likelihood of each possible true/false outcome**. And that this needs to be done and written down prior to the decision. I know this today, but I didn't know it or do it at the time. The second is that circumstances do change, and that legitimate adaptations in the **weight of evidence** can and should be made – but using the same discipline as before. The third is that in the absence of either of those pieces of structure, human factors such as emotional commitment to helping patients, fear of becoming redundant, and organizational needs will trump any amount of scientific data or pre-existing policy.

6

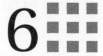

Safety Biomarker Development and Qualification in the Pharmaceutical Industry

Stephen T. Furlong

ASTRA ZENECA, WILMINGTON, DELAWARE, USA

One area of biomarker work in which there has been considerable interest and progress in recent years is safety biomarkers (SBM). Drug-induced organ toxicity is a major cause of attrition of late stage drug projects, and has also resulted in withdrawals of marketed drugs. One proposed means for improving the attrition rate is the development of improved SBM that enable earlier identification of organ toxicity. AstraZeneca has invested significant time and resource in SBM and much of my own work at the company in the last four years has been devoted to helping define what SBM are needed to support clinical trials, identifying assays that can be used for these new biomarkers, exploring how we can use these new markers to improve translational safety, and working with pre-clinical colleagues to help provide the clinical materials that will help enable SBM qualification. There has been rapid progress in developing new SBM, and exploratory studies on this topic are the subject of multiple consortia. However, significant challenges remain before these biomarkers can fulfill their promise. My vignette will describe the strategy we are using to pursue and qualify new SBM, some of the successes that we have achieved and challenges that remain for using these biomarkers to support clinical trials. In particular, there are several key challenges that we have been addressing in our work, namely identifying and collecting the appropriate human samples needed for qualification, characterizing pre-analytical and biological variability in these samples for selected SBM and developing the internal expertise to transition new assays to routine use for supporting clinical trials.

Before describing our experience with SBM qualification, it may be helpful to define how we use the term SBM. The definition of the general term biomarker, is well-established as:

> 'A characteristic that is objectively measured and evaluated as an indicator of normal biologic processes, pathogenic processes, or pharmacologic responses to a therapeutic intervention.'
> (Biomarkers Definitions Working Group, Clinical Pharmacology and Therapeutics 69 (2001), pp. 89–95).

The definition of an SBM, however, is less clear, and this lack of clarity has in some cases created some confusion and complicated the translation of promising biomarkers from

The Path from Biomarker Discovery to Regulatory Qualification. http://dx.doi.org/10.1016/B978-0-12-391496-5.00006-5

pre-clinical to clinical applications. In particular, pre-clinical SBM (usually thought of as biochemical biomarkers), are typically organ-specific biomarkers that are altered in response to *toxicological* doses of candidate drugs. The expectation is that elevations in these biomarkers will parallel changes in the histopathology of the target organ. Not finding elevation of such a biomarker generally provides support for moving a candidate drug into clinical testing. However, there are important distinctions between pre-clinical and clinical SBM. In particular, clinical SBM could be thought as biomarkers that inform about the lowest dose at which subtle, low-grade toxicities may appear. For any new clinical SBM there is the potential concern that the change in the marker in response to therapeutic dose of a drug may be too subtle to be of much value, or that there may be so much variability in the assay or 'normal' biological range that clearly demonstrating an effect related to organ damage may be almost impossible. Also, as opposed to pre-clinical use of an SBM, there is rarely (if ever) the option of correlating an elevation in the SBM with histopathology in clinical applications. Furthermore, translation of pre-clinical to clinical SBM can be thought of as potentially enabling two not so subtly different applications. The first is mitigating the population risk of drug-induced organ toxicity. The second is as a tool to improve patient safety in clinical trials and beyond by providing more sensitive tools for monitoring individual patients. Finally, in addition to biochemical biomarkers, there are a variety of genetic and electrophysiological tests, and imaging modalities, that could (and have been) referred to as SBM (see Table 6.1). For simplicity, in the rest of this chapter we will only consider qualification of biochemical SBM.

In thinking about the qualification of new SBM, we need to consider what traditional clinical chemistry tests these biomarkers would replace or for which they would be used as adjuncts. For example, liver function tests such as alanine aminotransferase (ALT) bilirubin, or kidney tests such as creatinine, meet just about any definition of an SBM when they are used in clinical trials to monitor for evidence of organ toxicity. These tests have been around for many years and the historical background of how these biomarkers came into general usage provides a useful context for gauging the difficulties of qualifying

Table 6.1   Uses for Safety Biomarkers (SBM)

SBM Use	Value Added
Identify safety failing projects early	Reduce level of uncertainty at key decision points
Identify compounds with weak safety profiles and elevated risk for causing future ADR, within a compound family early	Reduce level of late stage safety related attrition
Increase safety for trial subjects	Increased safety for trial subjects
Use common toxicity SBMs to monitor clinical trials and discover organ toxicity while damage is still reversible	Potential to stop safety failing projects early
Enable personalized healthcare	Enable launch of drugs that otherwise would have
Stratify patient groups based on their likelihood for adverse drug reactions (ADRs)	failed
	Enable more competitive launches

New safety biomarkers (SBMs) can add value in three areas. The emphasis of much recent work and the focus of the major consortia in this area has been on the first two applications. However, there are good examples (such as abacavir) that illustrate the potential of safety related assays to enable personalized healthcare.

new SBM to augment or replace them. Specifically, at the risk of belaboring the obvious, there is a major difference between the manner in which these biomarkers came into common use and the proscribed biomarker qualification process that is being advocated by both regulatory agencies and many in the biotech and pharmaceutical industries. Historically, there was no biomarker consortium to evaluate new test results, gauge their utility, decide when there is sufficient biological evidence to justify their broad use and provide recommendations on how to use the test. In the specific case of creatinine, for example, this analyte was first discovered in the mid-1800s and it took far more than a century before there was a test that was generally accepted as an assay for measuring kidney damage. There was no qualification process *per se* that resulted in this acceptance. Rather, there were many studies by many independent laboratories, with many patient samples, over many years. Eventually, a body of evidence built up that the medical and scientific community began to accept by consensus as an indicator of potential kidney damage. There was a similar history for ALT and bilirubin. In thinking about the history of how these older measures evolved, it raises the obvious question for me about whether we are being overly optimistic about how successful we will be in developing the next generation of biomarkers and how long it will take. Clearly there have been vast technological improvements in the recent past in our ability to discover and develop assays for new biomarkers. However, the recent history of consortia formed to qualify new SBM seems to be showing that, although there is good reason to expect some success, developing these new assays is likely to take far longer than initial estimates. Also, understanding differences between assays for the same SBM produced by different vendors, on different platforms (multiplex vs. single analyte assays, for example), and the biological variability inherent in healthy volunteer or different disease populations, to name just a few considerations, are key to having any likelihood of success in using these assays to support human clinical trials. As a result, at AstraZeneca we have developed a coordinated clinical–pre-clinical program designed to communicate with and contribute to external efforts to develop new SBM, while at the same time conducting internal activities with new SBM to ensure that we maximize the likelihood that these new assays can be integrated quickly into our clinical trial protocols.

With the considerations mentioned above in mind, one of the highest priorities for us on the clinical side of the company was to develop the company infrastructure for collecting human samples needed for SBM qualification. As shown in Table 6.2, it was clear to us early on (and paralleling efforts at other companies) that we would have the best chance of successfully qualifying new SBM by using a step-wise approach, beginning with establishing range and variation in healthy volunteers, followed by new SBM assessment in samples from patient populations, samples from patients treated with known organ toxicants and finally in samples from patients treated with our own candidate drugs. From the outset, our plan was to use these samples both for internal studies and also to share with external SBM consortia. In this regard, it has been truly surprising to me how complicated the seemingly simple and mundane task of sample collection can become when a key factor in the outcome of qualification studies is the criteria used to define the

Table 6.2 A Step-wise Approach to Establishing SBM Use

Sample Population Targeted	Output Data
Healthy volunteers	Range and variation in clinically normal individuals
	• Gender, age, ethnic variation
	• Intra/Inter patient variation
	• Longitudinal variation
	• Reference ranges
Disease groups (oncology, diabetes, COPD, etc.)	Range and variation in disease population(s)
	• Establish disease dependent changes
	• References ranges
Patient exposed to known toxicants Cisplatin – kidney Isoniazid – liver	Establish positive control
	• Tie to established drug-induced injury
Trial compound-specific	Early detection of safety signals
	• Create possibility for problem solving/clinical cutoffs

Understanding assay characteristics for a new SBM in well characterized human samples is an essential part of the qualification process. The type of data that can be derived from different sample populations is shown in the table.

needed samples. There is not space to treat this topic in depth here but three considerations that come up time and again include patient diagnosis, informed consents and use of retrospective samples. It is perhaps obvious that the way a disease population is defined will affect the results from studies using these samples. What may not be obvious is how complicated the discussions can become when cross-company consortia attempt to use samples from different studies with subtly different disease definitions, demographics, sample collection protocols and storage conditions. Similarly, trial subject informed consents routinely result in a 'gotcha' when attempting to use samples from more than one origin. Finally, on a not un-related point, most large pharmaceutical companies have large collections of patient samples that represent a significant company investment and which could represent a significant contribution in kind to consortia. In my experience, however, when and how such samples can be used is a subject of much debate, particularly when the samples were originally collected for reasons other than qualification of a specific SBM.

A second priority area for us, and a topic which I believe is key to effective use of a new SBM in our clinical trials, is a thorough understanding of the assay characteristics for the new SBM. This, again, is a very complicated topic, made no less so by technological considerations, biological factors, and financial considerations. Beginning with the financial, I once calculated that the cost to add a single new kidney biomarker assay to one of our large clinical trials would be approximately $25,000,000. No doubt some of our external partners would have been delighted by the prospect of the additional business. However, it would be irresponsible to add that much cost to a trial without first having fully demonstrated the value of the new assay. The area of SBM work that has continued to show the most promise is kidney biomarkers and this is an area where we are doing, and have done, considerable work to better understand the characteristics and value of these assays. Without describing all of the specifics here, with current technologies, it is not clear how easy it will be to clinically qualify a multi-analyte panel of new kidney SBM or how results from multi-analyte panels compare to those from single analyte assays. These comparisons are ones we are addressing. Furthermore, there are a host of assay parameters that must be explored before it is sensible to unleash a new assay on a large scale clinical trial. For example, just a few of the factors that can affect the results from a new assay include sample matrix (serum vs. urine vs. plasma), sample storage conditions and analyte stability under those storage conditions. Understanding inter-subject and intra-subject biological variability for a SBM or variability due to other factors such as gender, age or ethnicity is also a key consideration, and some of our initial work with new kidney SBM suggests that such variability may be high enough in typical trial subjects that it may be very difficult to be confident that an apparently elevated signal in an individual is actually correlated with, or a predictor of, organ toxicity. So although it may be tempting to apply an exciting new assay to a clinical trial, it is predictable that if some of the new assays are employed on a large scale without the type of groundwork described here, the result will be confusing and unsatisfying.

A third priority area for us has been to foster internal experience with new assays and to develop internal guidance for project teams wishing to use new SBM. It is probably obvious that introducing any kind of new assay into a clinical trial has the potential to cause major logistical and technical issues. Some of these issues can be the result of not fully understanding assay parameters and biological variability as described above. However, other problems can arise due to such mundane issues as poor communication with external vendors, sample shipping or storage problems, lack of agreed format for data transfer and a host of other details. As a result, an approach that we have tried to encourage is that conducting some type of small scale pilot(s) prior to moving into large-scale use of a new assay can eliminate unnecessary headache by identifying problems early. Potentially this can include working with more than one vendor to compare results, costs and ease of working and ultimately, can result in either formal or informal rec-ommendations concerning when to consider adding new assays, which assay protocols to employ, and which vendors to consider. Admittedly, for us, this is still very much a work in progress and has often been the subject of vigorous debate. However, as we have attempted to develop guidance for project teams relating to these new markers several considerations become clear. The first is that, as mentioned above, it is very easy to quickly inflate project team budgets by adding SBM or other biomarker work to trial protocols. For biomarkers qualified sufficiently that decision-making for a candidate drug is improved, the added expense can be justified. However, the examples where this is the case are, as of yet, few and far between. In fact, although it is often tempting to add a sexy new biomarker because of the excitement that such new technology generates, perhaps worse for the fate of a candidate drug than finding an actual 'wart' based on compelling but well understood data, is introducing uncertainty around a candidate drug project based on incompletely understood data from an exploratory biomarker. This risk is counter-balanced by the reality that ultimately the only real way for a team to begin to understand how to use a new biomarker of any sort is to use it and gain experience. Such experience gained and communicated through consortia can help, but does not substitute for actual hands on experience. As a result, my personal view (and the advice that I give project teams when asked) is that before adding an exploratory biomarker to a trial protocol one should be clear about how the data will be used. For late stage drug projects, it is hard to justify using a new SBM that is not thoroughly qualified. In earlier stage projects (e.g., Phase IIa) where the numbers of samples will typically be smaller and expense less it is easier to justify. An approach that one can use to further mitigate risk associated with using a new and incompletely understood biomarker is to include the new SBM in the trial protocol, and collect appropriate samples to carry out the assays. However, rather than immediately analyze the samples, one can store the designated samples for analysis at a later date. At that later date, the signal from traditional markers may be so clear that further data from the new biomarker will not provide any additional value. If, on the other hand, additional data is required to make decisions on a candidate drug, having these samples available could save the time and money that would be required to set up another prospective study.

In conclusion, biomarker qualification (or SBM qualification in particular), as a proscriptive approach to establishing the utility of a new clinical assay, is fundamentally different to historical approaches. Although biomarker qualification is the topic of many conferences, in the end what constitutes qualification is still a topic for debate and is dependent on the specific biomarker and context of use. What *is* clear is that developing data sets suitable to enable even internal decision-making requires considerable resource, and convincing the larger scientific and regulatory communities requires even more. In any case, a key ingredient to qualification of SBM for clinical use is the availability of appropriate human samples. Careful planning and choice of the most appropriate samples can greatly increase the likelihood for successful outcome of qualification studies. Finally, successful proscriptive qualification of new SBM will require cross-functional, cross-company and cross-agency cooperation at an unprecedented scale. Although there are already major consortia addressing this topic in both Europe and the US, how successful these consortia will be remains to be seen. With all the new technologies and new SBM assays that have become available in recent years, there is little doubt that some of these assays will ultimately prove their worth. The question is when?

7

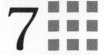

First-Ever Regulatory Biomarker Qualification – Review and Insights by a Participant

Frank Dieterle

NOVARTIS PHARMA AG, BASEL, SWITZERLAND

This vignette reviews the first successful formal biomarker qualification, focusing on the history of this qualification and on the best practices and lessons learned from this qualification of kidney biomarkers for pre-clinical and translational use.

Before this milestone of a first successful biomarker qualification with the health authorities, Novartis had a long history of biomarker development. Novartis biomarker research had not only focused previously on biomarkers typically used in early clinical studies, such as efficacy biomarkers, mechanistic biomarkers or stratification biomarkers, but also on biomarkers to monitor organ safety. In particular, internal biomarker research around chronic and acute kidney injury induced by overdosing immunosuppressant treatment regimens with tacrolimus or cyclosporine revealed a number of new, promising biomarker candidates to detect kidney injury early. For example, calbindin D28 was discovered as a renal protein biomarker by proteomic studies in animals treated with immunosuppressants [1]. However, a broader characterization and qualification of this biomarker beyond its specific utility of monitoring immunosuppressant-induced nephrotoxicity was not performed. In subsequent years, the introduction of toxicogenomics into pre-clinical research revealed a number of genomic biomarker candidates, such as kidney injury molecule 1 (KIM-1), clusterin, or lipocalin-2 (NGAL), which were modulated with kidney injury induced by various drug candidates. However, assays were not systematically developed to evaluate the performance of these biomarkers as peripheral biomarkers, as the general utility of these biomarkers in drug development was underestimated, since information about the potential of these biomarkers to monitor kidney injury and kidney diseases in humans was lacking at that time.

A turning point for safety biomarker development within Novartis was the announcement of the Collaborative Research and Development Agreement (CRADA) between Novartis and FDA [2]. The FDA–Novartis biomarker CRADA had three primary objectives:

1) To define a process for qualifying pre-clinical safety biomarkers for regulatory decision making.

2) To test this pilot process by submitting kidney-related safety biomarkers identified and characterized through pre-clinical studies to the FDA for qualification.

3) To propose how this process could be extended to qualify biomarkers for human use.

The processes developed in this collaboration laid the basis for the formal biomarker qualification process established by the health authorities Food and Drug Administration (FDA), European Medicines Agency (EMA), and Pharmaceuticals and Medical Devices Agency (PMDA). The qualification process, which has been published, covers the crucial elements to bring pre-clinical biomarkers forward to regulatory qualification [3]. Although nuances of the process have been changed during the first biomarker qualification (for example biomarkers are not qualified as general 'probable known biomarkers' but are qualified for a certain context of use), it provides guidance for generating appropriate data for pre-clinical biomarker qualification.

In the Novartis–FDA biomarker CRADA program the proposed biomarker qualification process was tested by following each element of the process map (Fig. 7.1) for the qualification of pre-clinical kidney safety biomarkers, which is described in the following. The selection of biomarker candidates was performed by an expert committee reviewing genomic biomarkers discovered in toxicogenomic studies, biomarkers from proteomic studies as well as biomarkers which have been published in pre-clinical and clinical contexts or which have been proposed in the context of human renal diseases. Biomarkers which were potentially translatable from animals to humans were preferred. In addition, biomarkers were selected such as to complement each other in terms of molecular processes as well as compartments of the kidney being monitored, with the ultimate goal of compiling a biomarker panel which covered all potential types of nephrotoxicity. In parallel, nephrotoxicants were selected with the goal of covering the most relevant types of drug-induced kidney injury, and applying to a wide variety of different modes of toxic action. This allowed the compilation of evidence about the utility and limitations of the biomarkers for as many drug classes as possible and removed limitations of only one specific type of kidney injury. Further, drugs which induced toxicity in other organs were proposed to evaluate the specificity of the biomarkers. Initially, 10 different known nephrotoxicants and two hepatotoxicants were proposed, which were evaluated in dose range finding studies. These studies were crucial to find the appropriate doses, administration route, frequency of dosing and duration of the main studies. A number of dose range finding studies were necessary to find appropriate study designs for the main studies and eight nephrotoxicants and two heptatotoxicants were finally selected for the compilation of study protocols for 10 pre-clinical studies. The protocols were jointly reviewed by a Novartis committee and FDA representatives. As shown in the scheme of the generic study design (Fig. 7.2), each study consisted of several dose groups and several termination time points per dose-group. This study design allowed: 1) the correlation of biomarker levels to different severities of injury, and 2) an investigation on whether biomarker changes can be detected prior to changes in histopathology and clinical parameters or at dose levels when histopathology and clinical parameters cannot capture drug-induced kidney injury.

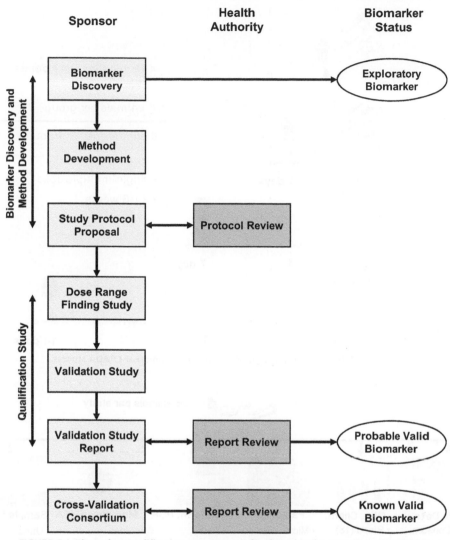

FIGURE 7.1 Biomarker qualification process map developed in the FDA–Novartis CRADA.

Since the requirements for biomarker qualification of kidney biomarkers were vague at the time when the studies were designed, an extensive number of parameters beyond the urinary biomarkers of interest were assessed in these studies, including in-life observations, an extensive panel of clinical parameters in urine and blood, genomic investigations for the biomarkers of interest and quantifications of protein levels of the biomarkers in blood and in the kidney in addition to the biofluid of interest. These extensive investigations allowed a very good mechanistic understanding of the biomarkers to be developed, including their journey from gene expression in the kidney, via translation into protein, secretion of the protein into blood, to excretion via urine.

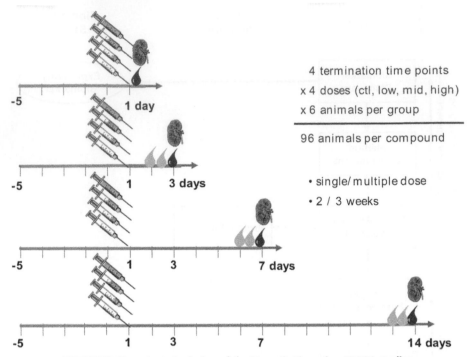

FIGURE 7.2 Generic study design of the Novartis Biomarker CRADA studies.

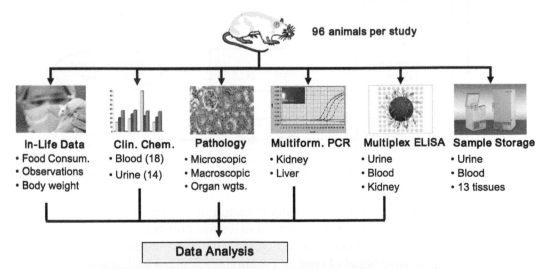

FIGURE 7.3 Parameters assessed in the Novartis Biomarker CRADA studies.

In addition, these extensive analyses also allowed an investigation of the organ-specificity of the biomarkers. As the first biomarker qualification for kidney biomarkers was completed, we were able to determine which parameters were critical for a successful qualification. Future biomarker studies may be conducted with a smaller number of parameters, reducing study costs significantly. For example, the biomarker qualification results showed that no systematic investigation for the protein biomarkers of interest on a genomic level was required. Also, measurements of protein levels in organs and blood were not required for the urinary kidney biomarkers. Finally, these results showed that the set of clinical chemistry parameters can be reduced to a panel of parameters monitoring the organ toxicity of interest only, and on a case-by-case basis potential other target organs specific to the drug employed.

To facilitate additional investigations, it is highly recommended to store tissue of critical organs, urine and blood in deep freezers. This approach allows leaner studies to be conducted, which will lower the bar of running specific biomarker qualification studies in industry and academia.

Within 18 months, the Novartis CRADA project successfully completed all the required dose range finding studies and 10 biomarker qualification studies. The result looked very convincing for a set of biomarkers and a submission of these biomarkers data package to FDA might have yielded a qualification of these biomarkers as 'probable known biomarker'. However, at this time the Predictive Safety Testing Consortium (PSTC) was founded as part of the FDA Critical Path Initiative. The goal of the PSTC is the collection of biomarker data from different participating pharmaceutical companies and the compilation of enough evidence of strengths and limitations of safety biomarkers for a formal submission to regulatory authorities for biomarker qualification. The initial focus of the PSTC was toxicities in kidney, liver, vascular injury and carcinogenicity, and the compilation of pre-clinical data to support pre-clinical safety assessment and enable the translation of drugs into humans. Novartis decided to join the PSTC and to share the results of the CRADA project within the consortium, as organ safety and safety biomarkers are generally seen as pre-competitive concerns in pharmaceutical companies and as the combination of data from different companies could further strengthen biomarker qualification packages and could result in a qualification of these biomarkers as 'known valid biomarkers'.

When reviewing the data from different member companies of the consortium, it became obvious that a number of companies had generated very similar data. For example for the kidney biomarkers, Merck, Pfizer and Sanofi Aventis, had also run a number of biomarker studies in rats. In particular, Novartis and Merck had very similar study designs and investigated an overlapping set of biomarkers. However, initially it was not clear how the data should be analyzed, how these analyses could be standardized, and how the results should be interpreted. Therefore, a series of face to face meetings and teleconferences took place to review various aspects of the datasets, such as histopathology assessments, specific details of kidney injuries observed, assays and analytical validation data, and different ways to analyze and represent the data and results. In these meetings a number of decisions were made to render the submission package to the health authorities as homogenous as possible:

• Histopathology: since histopathology assessment is the gold standard for pre-clinical biomarker qualification, it was considered as one of the most important aspects for success. To ensure reproducibility between studies from different member companies a common lexicon for histopathology assessment was crucial, which was compiled by the pathologists from the different member companies. The lexicon was compiled in a hierarchical structure starting with different processes of injury and recovery (e.g., necrosis, apoptosis, inflammation, basophilia...) at the highest level and covering the anatomical structures of the kidney in the next level ranging from a very broad integration in the second level (e.g., tubules) to a very fine partitioning in the subsequent levels (e.g., S3 segment of the tubules). This hierarchical approach allows injury to be characterized at different integration levels. Since some biomarkers are specific for certain types of injury occurring at a specific compartment of the kidney, while other biomarkers cover a very broad spectrum of pathologic processes not bound to one specific structure of the kidney, an exact match of biomarkers and histopathology at the same integration level is needed and can be allowed by this lexicon. For legacy studies, the slides had to be re-read by the pathologists using this standardized lexicon.

- Pre-processing of biomarker data: To account for the different dilutions of urine, it was decided to normalize the urinary biomarker concentration to the concentration of urinary creatinine similar to best practices of other urinary parameters in clinical chemistry. Although urinary creatinine can be down-regulated by severe kidney injury, it was considered non-problematic for those types of biomarkers which show increased urinary levels upon injury. However, biomarkers with down-regulated urinary concentrations upon kidney injury (for example TFF3) should be reported with and without creatinine normalization, as the normalization may mask the modulation of these kidney biomarkers. Further, it was decided to report and analyze all biomarker data only as fold-changes of the biomarker concentrations versus the average of biomarker concentrations for the matched control group. Using fold-changes versus absolute values allows accounting for differences in absolute concentration values reported by different assays. The PSTC decided to use the average value of the matched control value and not to use pre-treatment values of individual animals to prevent the introduction of additional variability.

- Further, the PSTC decided to use Receiver Operating Characteristic (ROC) as primary data analyses for the data [4]. For this purpose, histopathology is used as a binary variable (presence or absence of injury) and thresholds for the biomarkers are systematically varied while evaluating sensitivity and specificity. Then, sensitivity versus 1-specificity is plotted and the area under the curve (AUC) is evaluated. The AUC (1 for ideal biomarkers, 0.5 for a random estimator such as flipping a coin) is a measure for the diagnostic performance of a biomarker independent from selecting specific sensitivity-specificity combinations. The PSTC decided to use consistent thresholds for the tubular and glomerular biomarker sensitivity and specificity and to compare the different thresholds between different sets of studies. However, the overall performance of the biomarkers was judged and compared to the current clinical standards of serum creatinine and blood urea nitrogen (BUN) solely on the basis of the AUCs of the ROCs.

- Context of use: Based on the results of the biomarkers, the PSTC and the health authorities agreed that for each biomarker a context of use should be defined instead of an all or nothing qualification. In this case, the context of use describes the observed performance of the biomarkers including their strengths and limitations, the strengths and limitation of the data forming the qualification package, and the proposed context how these biomarkers will be used for drug development upon qualification.

Based on the results of studies from Novartis, Merck, Harvard Medical School and FDA laboratories, a package for seven biomarkers was submitted to FDA and EMA on June 15, 2007. Following the initial submission, a number of meetings and teleconferences were organized for clarifications and to discussion of open questions and additional analyses. In total, nine subsequent submissions were performed containing the results of additional analyses and of additional data. The discussions and additional analyses focused on two topics:

- Prodromal biomarkers: Some of the biomarkers were increased in animals treated with low doses of nephrotoxic drugs and/or at early timepoints under conditions where a standard histopathology assessment in these animals could not find lesions in the kidney. The PSTC claimed that the biomarkers were more sensitive and could be detected earlier than histopathology and track prodromal nephrotoxicity. Consequently, these animals and biomarker data were removed from the initial analyses of the PSTC, since it was unresolved whether histopathology was false negative, the biomarker data were false positive, or the biomarkers were detectable earlier and with greater sensitivity than pathology. These analyses were called exclusion analyses. The resulting lower thresholds for predefined sensitivity/specificity values were considered to be more conservative than standard data analyses, which for all these animals (biomarker-positive, histopathology-negative) biomarker results were considered as being false positive (inclusion analyses). The PSTC and the health authorities agreed to perform and review both analyses, concluding that, for a prodromal claim within a biomarker qualification, additional specific studies needed to be performed.
- Further, the health authorities requested a second blinded assessment of histopathology to evaluate the reproducibility of the assessment of the gold standard. To reduce the burden and costs implied by the re-reading of all slides, it was agreed to evaluate the reproducibility of histopathology only on a few selected slides.

The successful qualification of the kidney biomarkers, which was announced on June 12, 2008, was considered a major milestone by the PSTC, by pharmaceutical companies, and by the regulators as well [5]. Finally, a new process had been established as to how biomarkers can be qualified as enabling tools for drug development. This opened the door not only for developing and qualifying safety biomarkers for other organs and toxicities, but also for extending the qualified context of use of the kidney biomarkers beyond the original approved context (e.g., for late phase clinical studies).

The successful qualification has also helped to boost the use of the kidney biomarkers in drug development. This leads not only to a rapid increase in the amount of further evidence regarding the strengths and limitations of the kidney biomarkers, but ultimately also supports the development of drugs for unmet medical needs, which might not have been evaluated and developed in humans since an observed pre-clinical nephrotoxicity might have been considered unmanageable without kidney biomarkers.

References

[1] Steiner S, Aicher L, Raymackers J, Meheus L, Esquer-Blasco R, Anderson NL, et al. Cyclosporine a decreases the protein level of the calcium-binding protein calbindin-D 28kDa in rat kidney. Biochem Pharmacol 1996;51:253–8.

[2] PharmTimes Online, Safety biomarkers advance with completion of FDA–Novartis CRADA: http://www.pharmatimes.com/Article/08-03-31/Safety_biomarkers_advance_with_completion_of_FDA-Novartis_CRADA.aspx. Accessed June 17, 2013.

[3] Goodsaid F, Frueh F. Process map proposal for the validation of genomic biomarkers. Pharmacogenomics 2006;7:773–82.

[4] Wikipedia, Receiver operating characteristic: http://en.wikipedia.org/wiki/Receiver_operating_characteristic. Accessed June 17, 2013.

[5] FDA Press release, June 12 2008: http://www.fda.gov/NewsEvents/Newsroom/PressAnnouncements/2008/ucm116911.htm. Accessed June 17, 2013.

8

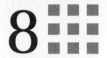

Metabolomics-Derived Biomarkers of Drug-Induced Skeletal Muscle Injury and Urinary Bladder Transitional Cell Carcinoma in Rats

Bruce D. Car, Donald G. Robertson

PHARMACEUTICAL CANDIDATE OPTIMIZATION, BRISTOL-MYERS SQUIBB, INC., PRINCETON, NEW JERSEY, USA

Metabolomic Biomarker for Drug-Induced Skeletal Muscle Injury in Rats

As pharmaceutical targets increasingly involve chronic conditions and inhibitors of a broader class of molecular targets in cell signaling, cell fate, and regulatory pathways, skeletal muscle toxicity is becoming a more important and common finding in the development of novel drugs. Creatine phosphokinase (CK) and aspartate amino transferase (AST) are typically used as clinical chemistry markers for skeletal muscle injury. They are, however, limited in terms of their sensitivity and specificity, particularly in rats. Newer markers, such as skeletal muscle troponin (sTnI), myosin light chain 3 (Myl3) and fatty acid binding protein 3(fabp3) are being developed to fill the need for better diagnosis of myopathies, but they have not yet gained wide acceptance.

To identify potential novel biomarkers of skeletal muscle toxicity, a metabolomics evaluation was conducted in a cerivastatin rat model. Drug-related myopathies occur with some frequency in rodents [1]. In rats, CK is a particularly poor biomarker, and AST, unlike in man, has a much shorter serum half life and is therefore less sensitive. Cerivastatin administered orally at 1 mg/kg/day in female Sprague-Dawley rats reproducibly produces a myopathy of type 2 muscle fibers within 14 days. Detailed nuclear magnetic resonance (NMR) analysis of urine from this model revealed that urinary concentrations of acetylated 1- and 3-methylhistidine (1MH and 3MH) consistently increased with the onset of the myopathy. Further analytical work identified a sensitive gas chromatography-mass spectrometry (GCMS) method for routine measurement of the isomers in both serum and urine. The two isomers of methylhistidine have long been studied as markers of muscle protein turnover [2]. 1-MH is a component of anserine (β-alanyl-1-MH), which is found in the cytoplasm of skeletal muscles in millimolar concentrations and 3-MH is a post-translational modification of myofibrillar actin and fast-twitch myosin in all species.

Despite their use as markers of muscle turnover, their use as markers of skeletal muscle toxicity had not been explored. While 3MH has broader cross-species application, 1MH appears particularly sensitive in the rat. Both increased and decreased urinary concentrations of methylhistidines are equally informative of isoproterenol-induced toxicity and muscle hypertrophy, respectively. Cerivastatin-induced myopathy of type 2 muscle fibers caused increases in urinary acetylated 1- and 3-methylhistidine which correlated with histopathologic findings [3,4]. In additional experiments with different myopathic agents, the increased urinary concentrations of 1MH and 3MH have been shown to be both sensitive and specific to the detection of relatively mild drug-induced myopathic injury. These data provided the empirical basis which justifies the use of these biomarkers for internal decision making in lead compound selection.

The broader use of these biomarkers in humans rather than rats is less promising given the highly variable meat consumption in man. Use of 1MH and 3MH addresses a significant deficiency in rats relative to the utility of CK and therefore provides clear benefit in non-clinical drug safety assessment and discovery counter screens for compounds with myopathic liabilities.

Metabolomic Biomarker for Causation of Bladder Tumorigenesis in Rats

Peroxisomal proliferator activating receptors (PPARs) are nuclear hormone receptors targeted for therapeutic modulation in diabetes. Findings with this class of molecules in two year rodent carcinogenicity studies, including hemangiosarcoma, liposarcoma, and urinary bladder transitional cell carcinoma have generally eluded comprehensive human risk assessment. With widespread distribution of PPARα and PPARγ receptors in tissues, including those transformed in carcinogenesis, separation of the role of the agonism from tumor development is unclear.

The following biomarker vignette derived from the carcinogenicity risk assessment of the oxybenzylglycine, nonthiazolidinedione PPAR α/γ agonist, muraglitazar [5–8]. An increased incidence of transitional cell papillomas and carcinomas of the urinary bladder were noted in rats at doses as low as eight times the projected human exposure at 5 mg/kg [6]. Papillomas and carcinomas were largely restricted to males and were predominantly located on the ventral bladder wall. Histopathology and scanning electron microscopy revealed early microscopic injury associated with the presence of calcium phosphate crystals. Increases in urinary pH were generally noted concomitant with crystalluria; a finding not consistently observed with different PPARα/γ agonists. The crystal-induced epithelial injury was hypothesized as causing epithelial cell death and regeneration. This was confirmed in BrdU-labeling experiments of the ventral bladder urothelium; a proliferative response strongly suspected in the genesis of tumor development. To determine the potential role of crystalluria in injury and carcinogenesis, crystals were solubilized in rats through urinary acidification with 1% dietary ammonium chloride. Urinary acidification of male rats dosed with muraglitazar abrogated crystalluria, early urothelial injury and cell proliferation (urothelial hyperplasia) and ultimately urinary bladder carcinogenesis.

To evaluate a potential role for pharmacology, the regulation of genes downstream of PPARα and PPARγ in the rat bladder urothelium was evaluated in the presence of muraglitazar-treated crystalluric and acidified diet, non-crystalluric rats. No changes in gene expression were observed, suggesting PPAR-mediated changes were not directly causative in urothelial profileration or carcinogenesis [5].

To evaluate the mechanism of muraglitazar-induced crystalluria and identify, if possible, a relevant safety biomarker, urine samples were collected from rats given muraglitazar for up to two weeks duration for metabolomic analysis. Following NMR spectroscopic evaluation of urine from treated compared to control rats, a striking reduction in divalent acid concentrations, including citrate and 2-oxoglutarate, was noted. Subsequent analyses of urinary citrate normalized to creatinine concentrations confirmed and extended these metabolomic findings. It was hypothesized that male rats experienced specifically decreased urinary excretion of divalent acids, in particular citrate, which contributed to a milieu highly permissive of calcium phosphate crystal formation. As these 'biomarkers' were considered likely mechanism-specific, further validation across species or with other agents that cause transitional cell carcinoma in rats was not sought. The likely specificity of the described mechanism of crystalluria with the corollary of urinary acidification ablating the precarcinogenic effect provided context for suggesting citrate as a biomarker for the specific potential of muraglitazar to cause bladder cancer.

To evaluate the potential risk of humans developing urinary bladder tumors, the urine from human patients treated with muraglitazar was evaluated for absolute excretion of citrate. The mechanistic rationale for the use of urinary citrate excretion as a biomarker was presented in the context of the limited validation provided above and accepted for single-time usage in human risk assessment. As reductions in citrate concentrations were not observed in muraglitazar-treated patients compared to placebo or pretest populations, it was considered unlikely that transitional carcinoma secondary to urinary crystallogenesis would occur in man. While citrate or other sensitive divalent urinary acid may be evaluated as a potential safety biomarker and possible explanation for nongenotoxic carcinogenicity with other agents, its potential use is likely very limited.

Summary

Metabolomics studies in rats established 1-methyl histidine and citrate as potentially useful, rat-specific biomarkers for skeletal myopathy and the causation of bladder transitional cell carcinoma, respectively. The first is a biomarker of injury and the second, putatively of pathogenesis, and therefore of potentially greater use in cross-species risk assessment.

References

[1] Car BD. Enabling technologies in reducing drug attrition due to safety failures. American Drug Discovery 2006;1:53–6.

[2] Jaweed MM, Ferraro TN, Alleva FR, Balazs T, Bianchi CP, Hare TA. Methylhistidine changes in tibialis anterior muscles of 6-mercaptopurine-treated rats. Toxicol Ind Health 1986;2:69–77.

[3] Aranibar N, Vassallo JD, Rathmacher J, Stryker S, Zhang Y, Dai J, et al. Identification of 1- and 3-methylhistidine as biomarkers of skeletal muscle toxicity by nuclear magnetic resonance-based metabolic profiling. Anal Biochem 2011;1(410):84–91. Epub 2010.

[4] Vassallo JD, Janovitz EB, Wescott DM, Chadwick C, Lowe-Krentz LJ, Lehman-McKeeman LD. Biomarkers of drug-induced skeletal muscle injury in the rat: troponin I and myoglobin. Toxicol Sci 2009;111:402–12. Epub 2009.

[5] Achanzar WE, Moyer CF, Marthaler LT, Gullo R, Chen SH, French MH, et al. Urine acidification has no effect on peroxisome proliferator-activated receptor (PPAR) signaling or epidermal growth factor (EGF) expression in rat urinary bladder urothelium. Toxicol Appl Pharmacol 2007;223:246–56.

[6] Tannehill-Gregg S, Sanderson TP, Minnema D, Voelker R, Ulland B, Cohen SM, et al. Rodent carcinogenicity profile of the antidiabetic dual PPAR alpha and gamma agonist muraglitazar. Toxicol Sci 2007;98:258–70.

[7] Waites CR, Dominick MA, Sanderson TP, Schilling BE. Non-clinical safety evaluation of muraglitazar, a novel PPAR alpha/gamma agonist. Toxicol Sci 2007;100:248–58.

[8] Dominick MA, White MR, Sanderson TP, Van Vleet T, Cohen SM, Arnold LE, et al. Urothelial carcinogenesis in the urinary bladder of male rats treated with muraglitazar, a PPAR alpha/gamma agonist: Evidence for urolithiasis as the inciting event in the mode of action. Toxicol Pathol 2006;34: 903–20.

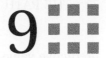

9

Molecular Biomarkers for Patients with Castration-Resistant Prostate Cancer: Validating Assays Predictive of Tumor Response

Daniel C. Danila[1], Howard I. Scher[2]

[1]*DEPARTMENT OF MEDICINE, WEILL CORNELL MEDICAL COLLEGE, NEW YORK, USA,*
[2]*MEMORIAL SLOAN-KETTERING CANCER CENTER, NEW YORK, USA*

Unmet Needs to be Addressed with Biomarkers

Critical to drug development in prostate cancer, as well as other tumor types, is the development of intermediate endpoints that can predict – dependably and early in the disease process – important clinical outcomes such as response to a specific treatment and survival time [1]. The heterogenous clinical characteristics of prostate cancer make a reliable assessment of clinical response to a specific treatment difficult, given that prostate-specific antigen (PSA) is not a validated surrogate of patient benefit or survival, that changes in radionuclide bone scans are difficult to quantify objectively or interpret, and that the Response Evaluation Criteria in Solid Tumors (RECIST) do not address how to assess changes in osseous disease, the most common site of metastatic spread [2]. Incorporation of relevant biomarkers into all phases of clinical testing is essential to accelerate drug development in this field [3].

Unfortunately, our ability to profile recurrent metastatic prostate cancers is limited because of the low diagnostic yield and the significant distress to patients of repeated biopsies of metastatic bone tumors [1]. As only a subset of patients may benefit from a treatment, even when a treatment target is present, blood-based assays are urgently needed to provide this information consistently and with minimal patient discomfort. The latter is particularly important in the management of prostate cancer, because the factors contributing to tumor cell growth and survival change over time as a result of the intrinsic biology of the tumor and the selective pressure of any prior systemic therapies that a patient has received [4].

Circulating tumor cells (CTC) are shed into the peripheral circulation from both the primary tumor and from metastases. Because they retain the intrinsic properties of the tumor, distinct from extent of disease, they have the same potential prognostic and predictive value of sensitivity to targeted therapies. However, according to the Oncology Biomarker Qualification Initiative road map, before the clinical utility of CTC biomarkers can be studied, it is first necessary to develop robust assays that can measure molecular biomarkers within the captured and/or isolated CTC. A formal biomarker qualification review process was recently introduced by the United States Food and Drug Administration (FDA). Biomarker qualification is a decision that, within the stated context of use, the results of biomarker assessment of a patient can be relied upon to have a specific interpretation and meaning in drug development and medical decision-making. The regulatory implication is that once the biomarker is qualified, drug developers will be able to use it in Investigational New Drug and New Drug Application/Biologic License Application submissions without requesting that the relevant FDA review group reconsider and reconfirm the suitability of that biomarker for each new drug [5,6].

FDA-Approved Method and Demonstrated Use

At some point in the development of a malignancy, cells detach from the primary tumor and invade, disseminate, colonize, and proliferate in distant sites. CTCs are rare, representing only a small proportion of cells in the circulation. Numerous techniques to isolate and capture CTCs have been reported, but only one method, CellSearch (Veridex LLC, Raritan, NJ), is analytically valid [7] and has been formally cleared by the FDA as an aid in the monitoring of patients with metastatic breast [8–11], colorectal [12,13], or prostate cancer [14–16].

It is now widely recognized that CTCs are often present and detectable in men with castration-resistant prostate cancer (CRPC) [17], and they are highly correlated with patterns of tumor metastasis to bone and visceral (versus lymph node) disease but only modestly correlated with measurements of tumor burden [16,18]. There is also evidence that CTC number is associated with overall survival (OS), both pre- and post-treatment, in metastatic CRPC [14–16,19–21]. These studies demonstrate that evaluation of CTCs at any time during the course of the disease allows for assessment of patient prognosis and is predictive of OS. As a result of these studies, we entered into a formal collaboration with the Biomarker Qualification Review Team at the FDA, with the goal of generating evidence to qualify CTC number assessed using the Veridex Cell-Search assay, as an efficacy-response biomarker/surrogate marker of OS in CRPC. This initiative, if successful, will enable better, faster, and less expensive drug development for the treatment of patients with this disease. To do so, we have prospectively embedded changes in CTC enumeration as a secondary endpoint in ongoing phase 3 trials of abiraterone acetate plus prednisone (trial registration ID: NCT00638690) [21] and enzalutamide (MDV3100; trial registration ID: NCT00974311) in men with CRPC progressing after treatment with docetaxel-based chemotherapies. The preliminary analysis of the Cougar AA-301 abiraterone study, showed that post-treatment CTC number was strongly associated with overall survival, and that the treatment effect on survival was explained using a biomarker panel that included CTC number and lactate dehydrogenase (LDH) [21].

Emerging Molecular Biomarkers

Both abiraterone, an inhibitor of androgen synthesis [22–24], and enzalutamide, a novel androgen receptor (AR) antagonist selected for activity in prostate cancer model systems with overexpressed AR [25,26], target the androgen signaling axis. The rationale for developing novel AR-directed therapies for CRPC came from molecular profiling studies showing that restored AR signaling is a consistent feature of CRPC [27], in part through AR overexpression and also through overexpression of androgen synthetic enzymes leading to increased intratumoral androgen levels [28,29]. Both of these alterations represent oncogenic changes in the tumor itself. Notable is that both agents have shown activity in patients post-chemotherapy, a point in the illness where the use of hormonal agents is typically not considered; this activity included dramatic PSA declines with durable radiographic control in some patients, though a distinct cohort of patients was intrinsically resistant. Of the patients who did respond, all eventually progressed, indicating acquired resistance to treatment. This highlights the need for predictive markers of sensitivity that can identify patients more likely to respond to targeted therapies and help us better understand the molecular mechanisms of resistance.

Genome-wide studies of tumors obtained from patients with prostate cancer reveal that the most frequent abnormalities relate to copy number alterations (due to gains and losses of specific genomic regions) rather than point mutations [30–32]. Indeed, the common oncogene mutations are rarely present in patients with prostate cancer. The phosphatidylinositide 3-kinases (*PI3K*) and AR pathways are the two most frequently altered pathways in prostate cancer. The phosphatase and tensin homolog (*PTEN*) deletion, most commonly by homozygous loss, is the most common mechanism of PI3K pathway activation, and is present in approximately 40% of primary tumors. AR gene amplification, a well-established genomic alteration present in approximately 50% of CRPCs, is not typically found at initial diagnosis. Accordingly, molecular correlates of response require direct analysis of tumor tissue obtained by re-biopsy at time of treatment initiation or from the original diagnostic sample. The success of the latter strategy depends on the concordance of the biomarker of interest at diagnosis versus relapse. A parallel approach that avoids this issue entirely is to molecularly profile CTCs obtained before treatment has begun. Multiple molecular profiling assays at the genomic, transcriptional, or translational level have demonstrated that CTCs isolated from patients at the start of treatment present a molecular profile very similar to that reported for late-stage tumors, suggesting that CTC analysis can be a noninvasive surrogate for routine tumor profiling (Fig. 9.1).

However, the validation of the molecular findings derived from laboratory studies on clinical specimens is limited by the difficulties in obtaining tumor tissue for profiling (both pre- and post-treatment), and by the lack of analytically valid assays for the predictive markers proposed. The Oncology Biomarker Qualification Initiative (a collaboration between the FDA, Centers for Medicare & Medicaid Services, and National Cancer Institute)

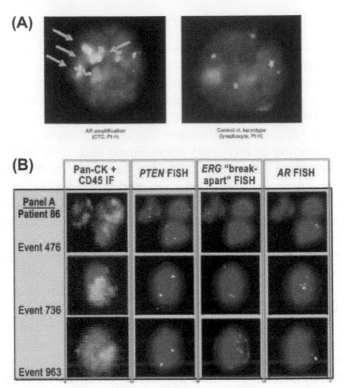

FIGURE 9.1 FISH analysis in CTC from patient with castrate prostate cancer, compared with the normal FISH signal in a leukocyte from the same sample. A) High resolution microscopy for CTC showing AR amplification (orange, arrows), with reference X centromere probe (aqua) and additional signals for ERBB2 (green) and 17 centromere (red). In comparison, normal leukocyte karyotype from the same patient is shown (adapted from Shaffer at al, Clin Cancer Research, 2007). B) FISH in Veridex chambers for CTC defined as CK (green) and DAPI positive, CD45 (red) negative immunofluorescence staining. FISH for PTEN, ERG break-apart, and AR FISH in CTC from same patient shows the heterogeneity of AR, ERG and PTEN copy number, however all cells show loss of the 5′-ERG signal, suggesting fusion of TMPRSS2 with ERG secondary to deletion *(adapted from Attard et al., Cancer Research, 2009)*.

requires that the assays used to measure the biomarker be analytically validated in a sequence of trials to generate the evidence to support its use in the given context [33, 34]. Clinically validated predictive markers have the potential to impact patient management directly, and to provide insights that may aid the future development of more effective therapies for this disease.

Validating Genomic Biomarkers in CTCs

Currently, the focus is on biomarkers that have been associated with drug sensitivity or resistance in laboratory models. Among the candidate genomic alterations associated with response and resistance in prostate cancer is the *TMPRSS2-ERG* translocation, often caused by interstitial deletion of the intervening region between transmembrane protease, serine 2 (*TMPRSS2*) and *ETS* related gene (*ERG*) on chromosome 21. This fusion, present in approximately 50% (range 30–70%) of newly diagnosed prostate cancers [35–38], represents more than 90% of the identified erythroblast transformation-specific

(*ETS*) translocations. In experimental models, the *TMPRSS2-ERG* fusion has shown a limited role in prostate tumorigenesis [37]. In clinical studies, the presence of the fusion was associated with low-grade disease [39] but not with higher risk of biochemical recurrence, metastases, or death [37,38]. Resulting in the translocation of an AR-regulated *TMPRSS2* gene with the *ETS* family member *ERG*, this fusion has been predicted to contribute to androgen-dependent tumor growth [40], suggesting a possible role as a predictive biomarker of AR-targeted sensitivity.

In one study, *TMPRSS2-ERG* translocation, detected by fluorescence *in situ* hybridization (FISH) in CTCs from patients with chemotherapy-naïve CRPC, was associated with increased chance of response to abiraterone acetate, but this association was modest and observed only in patients with a > 90% decline in serum PSA level [41]. The homogeneity of *ERG* gene rearrangement status in the analyzed CTCs was consistent with available tumor biopsies, in contrast to significant heterogeneity of AR and *PTEN* copy number alterations, suggesting that *ERG* rearrangements may occur earlier in prostate carcinogenesis.

To confirm the association between fusion status and prediction of treatment response to abiraterone, we developed a sensitive multiplex PCR-based method to detect *TMPRSS2-ERG* fusion in CTCs enriched from patients with CRPC [42]. We validated analytically the performance characteristics of the assay, including determining the range of conditions under which it would give reproducible and accurate data (Fig. 9.2) [43]. This validation required rigorous performance of three steps, as outlined by a draft guidance issued by the FDA [34]:

1) Pre-analytical assessment of specimen selection, handling, processing, and storage parameters;

2) Validation of the analytical characteristics to meet Clinical Laboratory Improvement Amendments (CLIA) regulatory requirements: establishing inter- and intra-assay

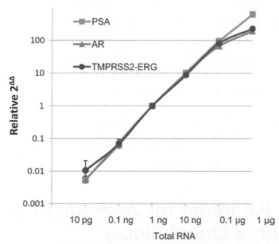

FIGURE 9.2 TMPRSS2-ERG fusion detected by reverse transcription polymerase chain reaction (RT-PCR) assay. Standard operating procedures included establishing the dynamic range of the sensitive multiplex assay for TMPRSS2-ERG, androgen receptor (AR), and prostate-specific antigen (PSA) genes. *Reproduced from Danila et al., Eur Urol, 2011.*

precision, linearity, analyte recovery, and standardization, and developing a comprehensive quality control program;

3) Establishment of post-analytical parameters for data management and storage.

Standard procedures were developed for specimen acquisition, processing, and testing using the validated TMPRSS2-ERG assay on a multiplex platform with intra- and inter-assay coefficients of variation required for performance in a CLIA-certified clinical laboratory. Although a PSA decline of $\geq$ 50% was observed in 47% of patients with the *TMPRSS2-ERG* fusion and 38% patients without, and post-therapy CTC counts of < 5/7.5 mL were prognostic for longer survival relative to those with CTC counts $\geq$ 5, *TMPRSS2-ERG* status did not predict either a decline in PSA or other clinical outcomes (Fig. 9.3) [42]. Interestingly, in both studies, there was significant discordance between *TMPRSS2-ERG* status in the primary prostate tumor tissue and in CTCs by FISH [41] or RT-PCR [42]. As also reported by others, this may reflect in part the multifocal nature of primary prostate cancers [44,45] and the inability to sample divergent clones in the primary tumor [46].

Although the two studies appear to be divergent, they both address the same gene target, but by utilizing different assays in different populations of patients: pre- and post-chemotherapy CRPC patients [41] compared to exclusively post-chemotherapy CRPC patients [42]. Also the correlation with a significant outcome such as OS is necessary to truly establish the clinical value of a biomarker. Further work is required to answer this question, but the early data establish that the impact of *TMPRSS2-ERG* fusion on response, if present, is modest at best.

Molecular Biomarkers in a CLIA-Certified Laboratory

Although these studies demonstrate the role of CTCs as surrogate tissue that can be obtained in a routine practice setting, current technologies to isolate CTCs have yet to mature sufficiently to enable the broad-scale genomic profiling studies that would be required to assess copy number alterations (particularly copy number loss) in the context of clinical trials. Problems with current technologies include the contamination of CTC samples with significant numbers of normal cells, and low CTC yields from many CRPC patients. A unique aspect of developing any biomarkers with clinical applicability is the effort to analytically validate the assay for use in a CLIA-certified laboratory, with established standards of assay performance and validation before clinical testing is initiated, and predetermined specimen acquisition, processing, and handling. This ensures the reproducibility and reliability of the biomarker data, but also enables early integration into clinical practice routines.

Changing the Paradigm for Assessment of Recurrent Prostate Cancer: a Liquid Biopsy

As noted, reliable measures are lacking to assess prostate cancer that has recurred after primary treatment are lacking. The development of molecular biomarker assays for CTCs

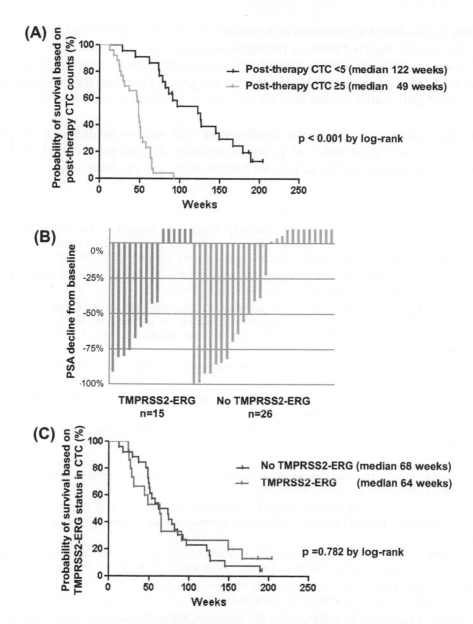

FIGURE 9.3 The role of CTC biomarkers in CRPC. (A) Patients with CRPC treated with abiraterone with unfavorable CTC $\geq$ 5/7.5mL at four weeks after therapy showed significantly shorter overall survival compared with patients with favorable CTC < 5 post-therapy (p < 0.001 by log-rank test); (B) waterfall plots showing PSA decline from baseline at 12 wk and TMPRSS2-ERG fusion measured by RT-PCR in CTC; (C) overall survival by TMPRSS2-ERG fusion status in CTC (p = 0.782 by log-rank test). *Reproduced from Danila et al., Eur Urol, 2011.*

is a step toward a 'liquid biopsy' that can profile an individual patient's cancer to guide the choice of treatment and understand why treatment has failed or is no longer working. This information, currently unobtainable for most patients with CRPC, could be extended to assessing outcomes for a number of other cancers. Exploratory studies are ongoing to prioritize biomarkers for evaluation in the stated context of use embedded in large clinical trials. The results reported here for *TMPRSS2-ERG* status in CTCs measured with a validated assay, and the sample size needed to detect a difference in survival, argue against further study of this biomarker alone in this patient group. However, the predictive utility of *TMPRSS2-ERG* status in combination with other biomarkers such as PI3K signaling activation status remains open [30,47–49]. The results also illustrate the importance of developing standards for biomarker development that include establishing the performance of the assay itself, followed by a prospectively planned sequence of clinical investigations that prioritize biomarkers for further study in large-scale trials.

References

[1] Morris MJ, Cordon-Cardo C, Kelly WK, Slovin SF, Siedlecki K, Regan KP, et al. Safety and biologic activity of intravenous BCL-2 antisense oligonucleotide (G3139) and taxane chemotherapy in patients with advanced cancer. Appl Immunohistochem Mol Morphol 2005;13:6–13.

[2] Scher HI, Morris MJ, Kelly WK, Schwartz LH, Heller G. Prostate cancer clinical trial end points: 'RECIST'ing a step backwards. Clin Cancer Res 2005;11:5223–32.

[3] Scher HI, Halabi S, Tannock I, Morris M, Sternberg CN, Carducci MA, et al. Design and end points of clinical trials for patients with progressive prostate cancer and castrate levels of testosterone: recommendations of the Prostate Cancer Clinical Trials Working Group. J Clin Oncol 2008;26: 1148–59.

[4] Scher H, Shaffer D. Prostate cancer: a dynamic disease with shifting targets. Lancet Oncology 2003; 4:407–14.

[5] Goodsaid F, Frueh F. Biomarker qualification pilot process at the US Food and Drug Administration. AAPS J 2007;9:E105–8.

[6] Goodsaid FM, Frueh FW, Mattes W. Strategic paths for biomarker qualification. Toxicology 2008; 245:219–23.

[7] Allard WJ, Matera J, Miller MC, Repollet M, Connelly MC, Rao C, et al. Tumor cells circulate in the peripheral blood of all major carcinomas but not in healthy subjects or patients with nonmalignant diseases. Clin Cancer Res 2004;10:6897–904.

[8] Budd GT, Cristofanilli M, Ellis MJ, Stopeck A, Borden E, Miller MC, et al. Circulating tumor cells versus imaging – predicting overall survival in metastatic breast cancer. Clin Cancer Res 2006;12: 6403–9.

[9] Cristofanilli M, Budd GT, Ellis MJ, Stopeck A, Matera J, Miller MC, et al. Circulating tumor cells, disease progression, and survival in metastatic breast cancer. N Engl J Med 2004;351:781–91.

[10] Cristofanilli M, Hayes DF, Budd GT, Ellis MJ, Stopeck A, Reuben JM, et al. Circulating tumor cells: a novel prognostic factor for newly diagnosed metastatic breast cancer. J Clin Oncol 2005;23:1420–30.

[11] Hayes DF, Cristofanilli M, Budd GT, Ellis MJ, Stopeck A, Miller MC, et al. Circulating tumor cells at each follow-up time point during therapy of metastatic breast cancer patients predict progression-free and overall survival. Clin Cancer Res 2006;12:4218–24.

[12] Cohen SJ, Punt CJ, Iannotti N, Saidman BH, Sabbath KD, Gabrail NY, et al. Relationship of circulating tumor cells to tumor response, progression-free survival, and overall survival in patients with metastatic colorectal carcinoma. J Clin Oncol 2008;26:3213–21.

[13] Cohen SJ, Punt CJ, Iannotti N, Saidman BH, Sabbath KD, Gabrail NY, et al. Prognostic significance of circulating tumor cells in patients with metastatic colorectal cancer. Ann Oncol 2009;20:1223–9.

[14] de Bono JS, Scher HI, Montgomery RB, Parker C, Miller MC, Tissing H, et al. Circulating tumor cells predict survival benefit from treatment in metastatic castration-resistant prostate cancer. Clin Cancer Res 2008;14:6302–9.

[15] Scher HI, Jia X, de Bono JS, Fleisher M, Pienta KJ, Raghavan D, et al. Circulating tumor cells as prognostic markers in progressive, castration-resistant prostate cancer: a reanalysis of IMMC38 trial data. Lancet Oncol 2009;10:233–9.

[16] Danila DC, Heller G, Gignac GA, Gonzalez-Espinoza R, Anand A, Tanaka E, et al. Circulating tumor cell number and prognosis in progressive castration-resistant prostate cancer. Clin Cancer Res 2007;13:7053–8.

[17] Danila DC, Pantel K, Fleisher M, Scher HI. Circulating tumors cells as biomarkers: progress toward biomarker qualification. Cancer J 2011;17:438–50.

[18] Shaffer DR, Leversha MA, Danila DC, Lin O, Gonzalez-Espinoza R, Gu B, et al. Circulating tumor cell analysis in patients with progressive castration-resistant prostate cancer. Clin Cancer Res 2007;13:2023–9.

[19] Olmos D, Arkenau HT, Ang JE, Ledaki I, Attard G, Carden CP, et al. Circulating tumor cell (CTC) counts as intermediate end points in castration-resistant prostate cancer (CRPC): a single-center experience. Ann Oncol 2009;20:27–33.

[20] Goodman Jr OB, Fink LM, Symanowski JT, Wong B, Grobaski B, Pomerantz D, et al. Circulating tumor cells in patients with castration-resistant prostate cancer baseline values and correlation with prognostic factors. Cancer Epidemiol Biomarkers Prev 2009;18:1904–13.

[21] Scher H, Heller G, Molina A, Kheoh TS, Attard G, Moreira J, et al. Evaluation of circulating tumor cell (CTC) enumeration as an efficacy response biomarker of overall survival (OS) in metastatic castration-resistant prostate cancer (mCRPC): Planned final analysis (FA) of COU-AA-301, a randomized double-blind, placebo-controlled phase III study of abiraterone acetate (AA) plus low-dose prednisone (P) post docetaxel. ASCO Annual Meeting, June 3–7, 2011; Chicago, IL; Abstract LBA4517.

[22] Danila DC, Morris MJ, de Bono JS, Ryan CJ, Denmeade SR, Smith MR, et al. Phase II multicenter study of abiraterone acetate plus prednisone therapy in patients with docetaxel-treated castration-resistant prostate cancer. J Clin Oncol 2010;28:1496–501.

[23] Reid AH, Attard G, Danila DC, Oommen NB, Olmos D, Fong PC, et al. Significant and sustained antitumor activity in post-docetaxel, castration-resistant prostate cancer with the CYP17 inhibitor abiraterone acetate. J Clin Oncol 2010;28:1489–95.

[24] de Bono JS, Logothetis CJ, Molina A, Fizazi K, North S, Chu L, et al. Abiraterone and increased survival in metastatic prostate cancer. N Engl J Med 2011;364:1995–2005.

[25] Tran C, Ouk S, Clegg NJ, Chen Y, Watson PA, Arora V, et al. Development of a second-generation antiandrogen for treatment of advanced prostate cancer. Science 2009;324:787–90.

[26] Scher HI, Beer TM, Higano CS, Anand A, Taplin ME, Efstathiou E, et al. Antitumor activity of MDV3100 in castration-resistant prostate cancer: a phase 1–2 study. Lancet 2010;375:1437–46.

[27] Scher HI, Sawyers CL. Biology of progressive, castration-resistant prostate cancer: directed therapies targeting the androgen-receptor signaling axis. J Clin Oncol 2005;23:8253–61.

[28] Scher HI, Kelly WK. The flutamide withdrawal syndrome: its impact on clinical trials in hormone-refractory prostatic cancer. J Clin Oncol 1993;11:1566–72.

[29] Holzbeierlein J, Lal P, LaTulippe E, Smith A, Satagopan J, Zhang L, et al. Gene expression analysis of human prostate carcinoma during hormonal therapy identifies androgen-responsive genes and mechanisms of therapy resistance. Am J Pathol 2004;164:217–27.

[30] Taylor BS, Schultz N, Hieronymus H, Gopalan A, Xiao Y, Carver BS, et al. Integrative genomic profiling of human prostate cancer. Cancer Cell 2010;18:11–22.

[31] Beroukhim R, Getz G, Nghiemphu L, Barretina J, Hsueh T, Linhart D, et al. Assessing the significance of chromosomal aberrations in cancer: methodology and application to glioma. Proc Natl Acad Sci U S A 2007;104:20007–12.

[32] Thomas RK, Baker AC, Debiasi RM, Winckler W, Laframboise T, Lin WM, et al. High-throughput oncogene mutation profiling in human cancer. Nat Genet 2007;39:347–51.

[33] FDA/NCI/CMS Oncology Biomarker Qualification Initiative. Memorandum of understanding between the FDA, NCI, and CMS for the FDA/NCI/CMS Oncology Biomarker Qualification Initiative. Document MOU 225-06-8001. January 2006. Last updated April 30, 2009. at http://www.fda.gov/About FDA/PartnershipsCollaborations/MemorandaofUnderstanding MOUs/Domestic MOUs/ucm115681.htm (accessed June 18, 2013).

[34] Center for Drug Evaluation and Research (CDER), Food and Drug Administration (FDA). Draft guidance for industry: qualification process for drug development tools. October 2010. at http://www.fda.gov/downloads/Drugs/GuidanceComplianceRegulatoryInformation/Guidances/UCM230597.pdf (accessed June 18, 2013).

[35] Tomlins SA, Rhodes DR, Perner S, Dhanasekaran SM, Mehra R, Sun XW, et al. Recurrent fusion of TMPRSS2 and ETS transcription factor genes in prostate cancer. Science 2005;310:644–8.

[36] Lapointe J, Kim YH, Miller MA, Li C, Kaygusuz G, van de Rijn M, et al. A variant TMPRSS2 isoform and ERG fusion product in prostate cancer with implications for molecular diagnosis. Mod Pathol 2007;20:467–73.

[37] Carver BS, Tran J, Chen Z, Carracedo-Perez A, Alimonti A, Nardella C, et al. ETS rearrangements and prostate cancer initiation. Nature 2009;457:E1; discussion E2–3.

[38] Gopalan A, Leversha MA, Satagopan JM, Zhou Q, Al-Ahmadie HA, Fine SW, et al. TMPRSS2-ERG gene fusion is not associated with outcome in patients treated by prostatectomy. Cancer Res 2009;69:1400–6.

[39] Fine SW, Gopalan A, Leversha MA, Al-Ahmadie HA, Tickoo SK, Zhou Q, et al. TMPRSS2-ERG gene fusion is associated with low Gleason scores and not with high-grade morphological features. Mod Pathol 2010;23:1325–33.

[40] Yu J, Mani RS, Cao Q, Brenner CJ, Cao X, Wang X, et al. An integrated network of androgen receptor, polycomb, and TMPRSS2-ERG gene fusions in prostate cancer progression. Cancer Cell 2010;17:443–54.

[41] Attard G, Swennenhuis JF, Olmos D, Reid AH, Vickers E, A'Hern R, et al. Characterization of ERG, AR and PTEN gene status in circulating tumor cells from patients with castration-resistant prostate cancer. Cancer Res 2009;69:2912–8.

[42] Danila DC, Anand A, Sung CC, Heller G, Leversha MA, Cao L, et al. TMPRSS2-ERG status in circulating tumor cells as a predictive biomarker of sensitivity in castration-resistant prostate cancer patients treated with abiraterone acetate. Eur Urol 2011;60:897–904.

[43] Pepe MS, Etzioni R, Feng Z, Potter JD, Thompson ML, Thornquist M, et al. Phases of biomarker development for early detection of cancer. J Natl Cancer Inst 2001;93:1054–61.

[44] Attard G, de Bono JS, Clark J, Cooper CS. Studies of TMPRSS2-ERG gene fusions in diagnostic transrectal prostate biopsies. Clin Cancer Res 2010;16:1340.

[45] Stott SL, Lee RJ, Nagrath S, Yu M, Miyamoto DT, Ulkus L, et al. Isolation and characterization of circulating tumor cells from patients with localized and metastatic prostate cancer. Sci Transl Med 2010;2:25ra23.

[46] Liu W, Laitinen S, Khan S, Vihinen M, Kowalski J, Yu G, et al. Copy number analysis indicates monoclonal origin of lethal metastatic prostate cancer. Nat Med 2009;15:559–65.

[47] King JC, Xu J, Wongvipat J, Hieronymus H, Carver BS, Leung DH, et al. Cooperativity of TMPRSS2-ERG with PI3-kinase pathway activation in prostate oncogenesis. Nat Genet 2009;41:524–6.

[48] Clark JP, Cooper CS. ETS gene fusions in prostate cancer. Nat Rev Urol 2009;6:429–39.

[49] Berger MF, Lawrence MS, Demichelis F, Drier Y, Cibulskis K, Sivachenko AY, et al. The genomic complexity of primary human prostate cancer. Nature 2011;470:214–20.

Toxicogenomic Biomarkers

10

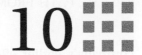

Gene Logic and Toxicogenomics Biomarkers

William B. Mattes

PHARMPOINT CONSULTING, POOLESVILLE, MARYLAND, USA

Gene Logic began operations in 1996 as one of the first companies to envision high quality gene expression data as a commercial resource. To this end it began with a marriage of its patented READS (restriction endonucleolytic analysis of differentially expressed sequences) technology [1], a differential-display based approach to monitoring changes in gene expression, with unique expertise in bioinformatics and database construction [2,3]. In January 1999, Gene Logic became one of the early adopters of the Affymetrix GeneChip® probe array, and began building its GeneExpress® gene expression database product using data from that system. In fact, Gene Logic worked closely with Affymetrix to refine procedures and analysis, as well as developing its own sample procurement and storage procedures, and the result was a premier, high quality, well annotated database of gene expression data from clinical samples. The resulting platform allowed, for example, both target discovery [4] and the investigation of tumor differences at the molecular level [5].

With the availability of genetic sequence information and tools such as polymerase chain reaction (PCR), by the mid 1990s the evolving field of 'molecular toxicology' included more investigations of the effect of toxicants on individual gene expression, particularly that of xenobiotic metabolizing enzymes such as the cytochrome P450s [6]. The concept of expanding such tools such as reporter gene assays to the screening of compounds for their effects on multiple genes [7] was commercialized by Xenometrix, Inc. [8], based in Boulder, Colorado. At the same time, microarrays based on cDNA were first described in 1995 [9], prompting Spencer Farr to establish Phase-1 Toxicology, with the goal of using gene expression, as monitored with microarrays, to assess a compound's potential for toxicity. By 1999 the field of 'toxicogenomics' was formally reviewed [10,11] (perhaps before any real data had been generated!), and in 2000 a report titled 'Toxicogenomics-based discrimination of toxic mechanism in HepG2 human hepatoma cells' was published [12], describing a microarray analysis of the effects of 100 compounds with various mechanisms of toxicity. Importantly, the publication highlighted the need for both the large number of compounds and the sophisticated informatics and statistical analysis for achieving meaningful results.

It was in this climate that Gene Logic hired Dr. Donna Mendrick in 1998 as Scientific Director (later Vice President) of Toxicology to develop a program of toxicogenomics. The

The Path from Biomarker Discovery to Regulatory Qualification. http://dx.doi.org/10.1016/B978-0-12-391496-5.00010-7
83

company's earlier efforts had focused on developing custom databases for individual customers. The business model going forward enlisted multiple customers in the collective development of a database sufficiently large and with diverse enough content to power statistical models that could predict the toxicity of a novel compound based on its microarray data. Already the power of a reference database of expression profiles had been demonstrated, not only in the work of Burczynski mentioned above [12], but also in the work of another microarray-focused company, Rosetta Inpharmatics, who demonstrated that hierarchical clustering of 127 experiments and 568 genes could identify temporal patterns of coordinated gene expression [13]. Yet both of these reports relied upon cell culture type experiments.

Several aspects of the Gene Logic toxicogenomics effort were novel, not the least of which was the concept of funding the development of a large database and predictive modeling system through partnerships with a number of pharmaceutical companies. However, this partnership extended beyond simple financial contributions, as a Toxicogenomics Database Management Committee (TDMC) of representatives from these companies provided scientific input into the design and capabilities of the database, and the goals of the predictive modeling system. At various times in the development of ToxExpress® database and ToxScreen™ models the partners included AstraZeneca, Biogen Idec, Boehringer Ingelheim, Daiichi Sankyo, Dainippon Sumitomo, Millennium Pharmaceuticals, Avalon Pharmaceuticals, Novartis, Organon, Pfizer, Sanofi-Aventis, Takeda and Wyeth-Ayerst. Quarterly meetings allowed for collective advice on compound selection and classification, study designs to be given, and importantly key elements of the goals and characteristics of the predictive modeling program could be discussed. In addition, bi-weekly teleconferences with one individual per customer were headed by Dr. Mendrick to ensure a close working relationship in this rapidly moving field.

While the word 'predict' means 'to declare or indicate in advance; especially: foretell on the basis of observation, experience, or scientific reason' [14], it does not have a simple, uniform definition in toxicology. In the practice of safety assessment in drug development, animal studies are intended to 'predict' toxicities that may arise during human clinical trials. Similarly, many *in vitro* studies with cultured rat cells are designed to 'predict' the *in vivo* toxicity of compounds [15]. A common theme is the desire to save money and time, and reduce the unnecessary exposure of either animals or humans to toxicants, by developing decision-enabling data earlier in the safety assessment process. The endpoints making up such data are actually 'predictive biomarkers'. And while the use of predictive biomarkers is attractive in principle, establishing confidence in their prediction is complicated by the stochastic process of disease and/or toxicity [16,17]. Surrogate endpoints in clinical trials are examples of predictive biomarkers that have in the past failed careful scrutiny [18]. In practice the acceptance of predictive biomarkers (or data) has much to do with the business process applicable at the time and the intuitive appeal to the decision maker. Thus, *in vitro* systems used for screening a series of compounds to predict 'toxicity' early in drug development do so at a point where little investment in any particular compound has been made, and by ranking, and not eliminating, compounds the criticality of the decision is limited. Likewise the prediction of rat renal pathology occurring after 28 days of treatment from kidney gene expression data obtained after five days of treatment represents an intuitive (and readily confirmed) approach [19]. However, the prediction of human adverse events from animal studies, despite its long history, continues to elicit controversy [20,21].

Yet in the early, 'heady' days of the 'omics revolution, there was wide speculation as to the capabilities of the technology and its potential in toxicology [22]. As noted above, global gene expression changes do precede overt morphological pathology for several types of toxicity. By extension, global gene expression changes observed early in a rat treated with a novel compound may be hypothesized to monitor molecular events that in humans could lead to adverse drug reactions. The TDMC embraced this hypothesis and thus the toxicogenomics program at Gene Logic was built on studies in rats treated with compounds known to elicit certain pathologies in rats as well as those that were known to elicit certain pathologies (e.g., hepatitis) in humans. In some cases the latter compounds were ones that had little evidence for eliciting a corresponding pathology in rats, i.e., these were deemed idiosyncratic, human-specific toxicants. Given the then recent withdrawals of several marketed drugs due to such 'idiosyncratic' liver toxicity, the major focus of the program was on hepatotoxic drugs, both those hepatotoxic across species and those human-specific, idiosyncratic hepatotoxins. The goal was to develop predictive models based upon gene expression that would identify early in development, indeed in very short term rat studies, the potential a novel compound had for causing idiosyncratic drug-induced liver injury in humans.

Wikipedia notes that the phrase 'the devil is in the details' comes from 'God is in the detail' and implies that it is the details that make for success or failure in an effort [23]. The details in the ToxExpress® database and ToxScreen™ models were indeed important, and were the matter for much discussion in TDMC meetings and among Gene Logic scientists and statisticians. One relatively noncontentious detail was the choice of target organs from which to collect gene expression data, and for which to develop predictive models: rat liver, heart and kidney. Other tissues (blood and bone marrow) were collected and stored to allow future gene expression analysis, and a considerable program was developed using cultured rat and human hepatocytes. In addition, data was acquired with canine liver, heart and kidney as well. Still, the focus for the major period of model development was the three organs mentioned first. Study design was guided by range finding studies to determine doses for test compounds that would elicit mild toxicity in the target organ within two weeks or toxicity in another organ, exaggerated pharmacology, or other clear signs of adverse reaction. This 'toxic' dose, as well as a lower, sometimes pharmacological, dose was used in the 'definitive' studies, where tissues were collected not only for gene expression analysis but also microscopic histopathology. Clinical chemistry data and hematology were also obtained from all studies, with all data being captured in the ToxExpress® database. The sacrifice time points were dictated by the desire to predict toxicity from early gene expression events, hence six and 24 hours after initial dosing, and then a later time point, determined from range finding studies, at which toxicity or pathology was noted by conventional end-points. Replicate animals were included in all groups, as well as time-matched vehicle controls.

The approach to the collection and modeling of gene expression data was also a detail that played an important role. First and foremost was the choice of the relatively new and expensive Affymetrix microarray technology. Gene Logic had partnered with Affymetrix to improve analysis techniques, but even so, most of the 'genes' represented on the available RG-U34 rat genome array were 'expressed sequence tags' (ESTs) representing mRNAs from as yet unknown genes. Even though a draft of the human genome was announced in 2000, and completed in 2003 and a draft of the rat genome was reported in 2004, annotation by homology to genomic DNA often shed little light on the biological role of many ESTs. It should be noted that even now the multiple roles that genes such as glyceraldehyde-3-phosphate dehydrogenase (G3PDH) play are still being uncovered [24]. For biologists and toxicologists accustomed to hypothesis-driven experiments, micro-array experiments produced a shocking deluge of undefined data. But given the belief that ESTs indeed had a yet undiscovered function, it seemed reasonable to include their re-sponses to toxicants in predictive models. This was an important cornerstone in the modeling approach that Gene Logic took, coupled with the development of models that eliminated 'genes' whose behavior did not contribute to accuracy.

The collective input of the TDMC was crucial in setting aspects of the predictive models. The 'paradigm' compounds chosen for study were done so after group agree-ment on the expected pathology the compound should produce and the value it would have for the overall model. The group input affirmed the decision to utilize all genes on the arrays in the pool for gene selection for model development; i.e., not to pre-select genes but allow the best markers to be identified. Coming from a pharmaceutical industry standpoint looking to advance compounds with potential, the directive was to formulate models with very low false positive rates. Finally the types of models pursued were a collaborative decision, albeit the final output was dictated by what models the data could robustly support: a model of 'general' toxicity, models of target organ pathology or mechanism, and then models comparing the behavior of the data of an unknown com-pound to the data associated with compounds in the database (compound similarity). The overall considerations, design, and validation of these models have been thoroughly described by Mark Porter in a 2008 retrospective [25].

While qualification and validation of biomarkers are discussed elsewhere in this book, validation of predictive models is generally considered a statistical problem [25]. For many predictive models being developed at the time, there was considerable debate as to the best approach; however, Gene Logic used a 'compound drop' technique, whereby an entire dataset was eliminated from the model, the model rebuilt, and the dropped dataset tested on the rebuilt model. This technique was affirmed by the TDMC partners, although it was understood that many of these companies would conduct their own tests of the database using internally derived data. In some cases these 'internal validation' studies were shared with Gene Logic and the other partners, but given the number of analyses

Gene Logic performed on blinded company data, it is hard to say whether some of these datasets represented internal validation effort as well.

As of January, 2006 Gene Logic had provided predictive profiles on > 400 customer datasets from 22 companies. Yet, in late 2007 Gene Logic's genomics business was purchased by an Indian company for a fraction of the cost of running studies, acquiring gene expression data, developing the database and models. Considering that the entire program was not only funded but designed by partner companies, one would think that it would have been successful. Business decisions aside, a system that promised to improve the drug development pipeline by preventing the development of drugs with adverse events surely should have had traction in the marketplace.

As noted above, it was clear that customers did carry out internal 'validation' exercises, but the feedback from such exercises was limited. One critical feedback came from a customer that had carried out the gene expression profile and application of ToxPredict™ predictive models on a number of early stage development compounds. The results for a number of the compounds indicated the potential for human hepatotoxicity. However, the conventional endpoints gave no indication of hepatotoxicity in the rats. The project team overseeing the compound's development concluded that there was no convincing evidence to halt development regardless of the ToxPredict™ results. In short, while the safety assessment thought leaders had accepted the cornerstone of the Gene Logic program, developing a system to predict adverse events in the absence of overt rat pathology, the overall decision makers in the company rejected it when faced with actually halting programs mid-development.

This anecdote highlights the difficulty of qualifying biomarkers when multiple and/or key stakeholders do not agree on the process of qualification. As noted above, qualification of predictive biomarkers or surrogate endpoints, is currently an onerous and contentious process. One might expect that qualification of a predictive biomarker that will halt development of a compound, has added difficulties due to the economic, organizational, and often personal drive to move compounds through the pipeline. Certainly the Gene Logic system, keying off of data from early rat studies, was entering the pipeline at a point when such drives can already be in place. Screens that 'rank' compounds at an earlier stage of lead optimization sometimes have wider acceptance.

Other factors also played into ToxPredict™ not seeing wider use. As noted, the system used a great number of marker genes and ESTs, and while statistically validated, the results were not easily fashioned into a mechanistic story. The conflict between using a larger number of markers, many of which have functions yet to be determined, and using a smaller number of well-understood markers has been discussed [25]. The statistical and biological (namely, the response of a gene with currently unknown function may later prove be more relevant to the biology) arguments for the former approach notwithstanding, many toxicologists needed to be able to provide a mechanistic explanation. Hence the many-gene-statistical approach was often labeled a 'black box'.

Another factor might be considered the NIH effect – Not Invented Here – as many companies felt that the internal development of a database and predictive system was more suitable to their organization. In some cases this might have come from the belief that using proprietary compounds created a database more relevant to their programs. The Gene Logic database certainly included diverse structures, but there is always the tension between the chemical viewpoint that chemical space is a critical concern and the toxicological viewpoint that certain pathologies and the molecular mechanisms that lead to them are limited in number and common to many different structures.

Ultimately there may be many reasons why the few commercial toxicogenomics 'biomarkers' failed to be widely accepted. Perhaps the key element as noted above was the lack of an open discussion in wider community as to what would constitute qualification for any given use. Added to this was the cost of the gene expression data; more successful toxicogenomics 'biomarkers' have been transferred to lower cost PCR screens [26]. Furthermore all predictive biomarkers suffer from the limitation that if decision makers ultimately discount their ability to halt a program they simply add useless cost (see Chapter 5).

There are lessons to be learned from the development of toxicogenomics biomarkers, but perhaps the most important is that they have not been widely discussed. Sadly, toxicogenomics is often considered a fad past its time. Worse, there are new fads that could learn from the lessons of toxicogenomics. As George Santayana wrote: 'Those who cannot remember the past are condemned to repeat it.'

References

[1] Lennon GG. High-throughput gene expression analysis for drug discovery. Drug Discov Today 2000; 5:59–66.

[2] Chen IM, Kosky AS, Markowitz VM, Szeto E, Topaloglou T. Advanced query mechanisms for biological databases. Proc Int Conf Intell Syst Mol Biol 1998;6:43–51.

[3] Eckman BA, Kosky AS, Laroco Jr LA. Extending traditional query-based integration approaches for functional characterization of post-genomic data. Bioinformatics 2001;17:587–601.

[4] Orr MS, Scherf U. Large-scale gene expression analysis in molecular target discovery. Leukemia 2002;16:473–7.

[5] Prakash K, Pirozzi G, Elashoff M, Munger W, Waga I, Dhir R, et al. Symptomatic and asymptomatic benign prostatic hyperplasia: molecular differentiation by using microarrays. Proc Natl Acad Sci U S A 2002;99:7598–603.

[6] Vanden Heuvel JP, Clark GC, Thompson CL, McCoy Z, Miller CR, Lucier GW, et al. CYP1A1 mRNA levels as a human exposure biomarker: use of quantitative polymerase chain reaction to measure CYP1A1 expression in human peripheral blood lymphocytes. Carcinogenesis 1993;14:2003–6.

[7] MacGregor JT, Farr S, Tucker JD, Heddle JA, Tice RR, Turteltaub KW. New molecular endpoints and methods for routine toxicity testing. Fundam Appl Toxicol 1995;26:156–73.

[8] Todd MD, Lee MJ, Williams JL, Nalezny JM, Gee P, Benjamin MB, et al. The CAT-Tox (L) assay: a sensitive and specific measure of stress-induced transcription in transformed human liver cells. Fundam Appl Toxicol 1995;28:118–28.

[9] Schena M, Shalon D, Davis RW, Brown PO. Quantitative monitoring of gene expression patterns with a complementary DNA microarray. Science 1995;270:467–70.

[10] Farr S, Dunn 2nd RT. Concise review: gene expression applied to toxicology. Toxicol Sci 1999;50:1–9.

[11] Nuwaysir EF, Bittner M, Trent J, Barrett JC, Afshari CA. Microarrays and toxicology: the advent of toxicogenomics. Mol Carcinog 1999;24:153–9.

[12] Burczynski ME, McMillian M, Ciervo J, Li L, Parker JB, Dunn RT, et al. Toxicogenomics-based discrimination of toxic mechanism in HepG2 human hepatoma cells. Toxicol Sci 2000;58:399–415.

[13] Hughes TR, Marton MJ, Jones AR, Roberts CJ, Stoughton R, Armour CD, et al. Functional discovery via a compendium of expression profiles. Cell 2000;102:109–26.

[14] Merriam-Webster. Predict – Definition and More from the Free Merriam-Webster Dictionary. Available: http://www.merriam-webster.com/dictionary/predict. 2012. Last accessed 1 August 2012.

[15] Waterfield CJ, Westmoreland C, Asker DS, Murdock JC, George E, Timbrell JA. Ethionine toxicity *in vitro*: the correlation of data from rat hepatocyte suspensions and monolayers with *in vivo* observations. Arch Toxicol 1998;72:588–96.

[16] Coggon DI, Martyn CN. Time and chance: the stochastic nature of disease causation. Lancet 2005; 365:1434–7.

[17] Cook NR. Use and misuse of the receiver operating characteristic curve in risk prediction. Circulation 2007;115:928–35.

[18] Psaty BM, Lumley T. Surrogate end points and FDA approval: a tale of 2 lipid-altering drugs. Jama 2008;299:1474–6.

[19] Fielden MR, Eynon BP, Natsoulis G, Jarnagin K, Banas D, Kolaja KL. A gene expression signature that predicts the future onset of drug-induced renal tubular toxicity. Toxicol Pathol 2005;33:675–83.

[20] Committee on Toxicity Testing and Assessment of Environmental Agents. Toxicity testing in the 21st century: a vision and a strategy. Washington, D.C: The National Academies Press; 2007.

[21] Olson H, Betton G, Robinson D, Thomas K, Monro A, Kolaja G, et al. Concordance of the toxicity of pharmaceuticals in humans and in animals. Regul Toxicol Pharmacol 2000;32:56–67.

[22] MacGregor JT. The future of regulatory toxicology: impact of the biotechnology revolution. Toxicol Sci 2003;75:236–48.

[23] Wikipedia_contributors. The Devil is in the details. Wikimedia Foundation, Inc; 2012.

[24] Dastoor Z, Dreyer JL. Potential role of nuclear translocation of glyceraldehyde-3-phosphate dehydrogenase in apoptosis and oxidative stress. J Cell Sci 2001;114:1643–53.

[25] Porter MW. *In vivo* predictive toxicogenomics. Methods Mol Biol 2008;460:113–43.

[26] Fielden MR, Nie A, McMillian M, Elangbam CS, Trela BA, Yang Y, et al. Interlaboratory evaluation of genomic signatures for predicting carcinogenicity in the rat. Toxicol Sci 2008;103:28–34.

11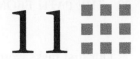

The When, Where and How of Toxicogenomic Submissions to Regulatory Agencies

The Deliberations of the HL7/CDISC/I3C Pharmacogenomics Data Standards Track 1 Toxicogenomics Working Group

Peter G. Lord

DISCOTOX LTD., HEBDEN BRIDGE, WEST YORKSHIRE, UK

Introduction and Background

In November of 2003, the Drug Information Association (DIA), United States Federal Drug Administration (FDA), Pharmacogenomics Working Group (PWG), Pharmaceutical Research and Manufacturers of America (PhRMA), and Biotechnology Industry Organization (BIO) organizations held a joint workshop to debate the use of pharmacogenomics in drug development and regulatory decision making. The main focus of the meeting was to review the 'Genomic Data Submission (GDS) Proposal' published November 2003 by the FDA (www.fda.gov/cder/guidance/5900dft.doc) subsequently replaced March 2005 by www.fda.gov/downloads/RegulatoryInformation/Guidances/ UCM26957. Following that conference, the Health Level 7 (HL7), Clinical Data Interchange Standards Consortium (CDISC), and Interoperable Informatics Infrastructure Consortium (I3C) organizations initiated a joint project to help build a consensus on the issues of pharmacogenomic data standards raised in the guidance document. Three sub-teams were formed, based upon the November 2003 Pharmacogenomics Standards Workshop, namely:

Track 1) Pre-clinical/Non-clinical Genomics (Toxicogenomics)
Track 2) Clinical Pharmacology
Track 3) Clinical Genomics.

The Track 1 Toxicogenomics Sub-team began in early 2004 by teleconference with eight representatives from the FDA and myself. I was the sole participant from industry.

Our first tasks were to appoint a sub-team leader (the author!) and to enlist more participants. The ILSI/HESI toxicogenomics committee [1] proved a good recruiting ground, and within a few months we not only had a regular and balanced group of attendees representing FDA and Pharmaceutical companies but also drew in representatives from United States Environmental Protection Agency (EPA), National Institute of Environmental Health Sciences (NIEHS), and European Federation of Pharmaceutical Industries and Associations (EfPIA). The participants are acknowledged at the end of this chapter.

Rather than consider microarray experiments from start to finish we decided to design some scenarios for hypothetical regulatory drug submissions in which microarray data would have been generated during the various stages of safety evaluation. This approach allowed us to not only avoid spending hours of discussion on how to standardize RNA extraction but also to consider the different purposes for which microarray data are put to use in pre-clinical drug development. It was not a simple matter to design case examples since at this time there was very little information available in the literature to base them on and the application of toxicogenomics in drug safety evaluation was still maturing. Three case examples were initially proposed, and all three proved their worth in driving the discussions. They illustrated the variety of purposes for which microarray data are generated in the drug development process from very early discovery stages through compound selection to the final stages of pre-clinical drug safety evaluation. By debating these different aims, the sub-team was able to address the fundamental question of how much information from a microarray experiment should be made available to assist a regulatory reviewer of a drug safety submission. Viewpoints on this ranged from: 'all toxicogenomic microarray data need to be submitted' – as for the submission of manuscripts to a scientific journal; to 'the submission of all microarray data is basically a data dump and only those toxicogenomic data directly relevant for the safety evaluation need to be submitted' – the emphasis here being that a safety case is primarily built on a synthesis to a subset of microarray data to formulate hypotheses. Consequently, it is more helpful for the reviewer to evaluate those data generated to test the hypotheses rather than the considerable amount of the data generated to arrive at those hypotheses.

Toxicogenomic Applications in Drug Discovery and Development

In the pharmaceutical industry, toxicogenomics is applied in two broad areas:

1. Predictive toxicology studies, aimed at providing comprehensive, comparative data related to toxic potential in order to make informed decisions on a drug's development.
2. Investigative toxicology studies, aimed at understanding the mechanism of toxicity of a drug in pre-clinical species in order to determine relevance to clinical use and possibly to identify a novel biomarker of toxicity.

In the first type of toxicogenomic application, predictive toxicology studies are not intended to provide information to directly support drug safety claims. Rather, they are performed to assess the likelihood of success in the development of a drug, or to aid in the design of subsequent pre-clinical studies. Regulatory studies provide the definitive testing of a drug's toxicity but can be carried out more effectively when they incorporate the testing of the hypotheses generated by predictive toxicology assays. Therefore, data from these preliminary studies are not expected to be included in a regulatory submission.

Investigative toxicology studies, however, are carried out with the intent of using the information from those studies to support a risk assessment and safety claim. Consequently, if DNA microarray experiments are incorporated into an investigative toxicology program, the gene expression data generated may be required for a submission.

An additional consideration is that during the drug discovery phase, microarray data may be generated to assess aspects of a compound's efficacy or pharmacological activity in model systems. These data may be mined proactively or retrospectively for potential safety concerns. However, the main purpose of generating the data is not toxicity evaluation; accordingly, such data may be considered to be unnecessary for inclusion in a regulatory submission.

After considering these different activities, the sub-team focused on investigative toxicology applications of toxicogenomics having direct relevance to regulatory drug safety evaluation. These are situations where microarray data submission is likely. The group developed two case examples, each drawing on information from the scientific literature and developed along the lines of investigative toxicology studies intended to support safety claims.

The Case Examples

The first case, describing a gamma secretase inhibitor, concentrated on data generated for hypothesis generation to explain a pre-clinical or clinical finding and/or to identify biomarkers of safety/efficacy. The second example based on a hypothetical hypolipidemic drug, addressed data generated for hypothesis confirmation supporting risk/benefit assessment.

A Hypothetical Submission in Support of the Safety Claims for a Gamma Secretase Inhibitor

Papers by Searfoss et al. [2] and Milano et al. [3] provided the basis for this example, both being studies of the pre-clinical toxicities of a gamma secretase inhibitors being developed for treatment of Alzheimer's disease. The toxicity of concern for this example is gastrointestinal pathology, characterized by goblet cell metaplasia accompanied by symptoms of severe diarrhea in pre-clinical animal species. Investigations of the toxicity would include comparative gene expression profiling experiments. These would be aimed at gaining an understanding of the molecular mechanism of the gastrointestinal (GI) toxicity in rats mediated by compounds of this class. The gene expression end points would also be used to understand and to further assess how mechanistically distinct compounds in development are in terms of propensity to induce GI toxicity, information

BOX 11.1 CASE EXAMPLE 1: TOXICOGENOMIC ANALYSIS OF THE γ SECRETASE INHIBITORS X, Y AND Z

BACKGROUND

Development of the γ secretase inhibitor compounds X and Y was halted due to severe but reversible diarrhea seen in the clinic, which may be due to the GI toxicity observed in rats and monkeys seen as goblet cell metaplasia. Compound Z has a more favorable safety profile in the rat and monkey. To further establish the clinical safety of compound Z, and to develop mechanism-based biomarkers to monitor for clinical safety, comparative toxicogenomic experiments were conducted.

RESULTS

Compounds X, Y and Z were profiled using comparative toxicogenomic experiments in rats. Compounds X and Y induced GI toxicity, while Z demonstrated no GI toxicity. Comparative analysis of the gene expression data yielded a list of dysregulated genes that can differentiate toxic and non-toxic compounds. From this set of genes, Notch signaling was identified as being significantly dysregulated. Amongst this small set of genes were adipsin and rath-1. Follow up studies on the behavior of protein products of these genes, using an ELISA approach, showed that these were induced in the GI tract and were found at elevated levels in feces of treated animals. Data from this and other follow up studies demonstrated the mechanistically based rationale for monitoring the protein level of Adipsin or Rath-1 in feces as biomarkers for GI toxicity mediated by inhibiting Notch signaling. This will assist with differential diagnosis of drug induced goblet cell changes and be useful for monitoring the safety of compound Z and other γ secretase inhibitors during clinical investigations.

CASE EXAMPLE 1: TOXICOGENOMIC ANALYSIS OF THE γ SECRETASE INHIBITORS X, Y AND Z

Background

Development of the γ secretase inhibitor compounds X and Y was halted due to severe but reversible diarrhea seen in the clinic, which may be due to the GI toxicity observed in rats and monkeys seen as goblet cell metaplasia. Compound Z has a more favorable safety profile in the rat and monkey. To further establish the clinical safety of compound Z and to develop mechanism based biomarkers to monitor for clinical safety, comparative toxicogenomic experiments were conducted.

Results

Compounds X, Y and Z were profiled using comparative toxicogenomic experiments in rats. Compound X and Y induced GI toxicity while Z demonstrated no GI toxicity. Comparative analysis of the gene expression data yielded a list of dysregulated genes that can differentiate toxic and non toxic compounds. From this set of genes, Notch signaling was identified as being significantly dysregulated. Amongst this small set of genes were adipsin and rath-1. Follow up studies on the gene products using an ELISA approach showed that these were induced in the GI tract and were found at elevated levels in feces of treated animals. Data from this and other follow up studies demonstrated the mechanistically based rationale for monitoring the protein level of Adipsin or Rath-1 in feces as biomarkers for GI toxicity mediated by inhibiting Notch signaling. This will assist with differential diagnosis of drug induced goblet cell changes and be useful for monitoring the safety of compound Z and other γ secretase inhibitors during clinical investigations.

that would support candidate selection. Finally, another output would be the identification of mechanism based protein biomarkers that enhance clinical safety monitoring of such compounds. Box 11.1 shows a brief description of this hypothetical case. In this example the microarray derived gene expression data, although needed to identify the safety biomarkers, are not needed to validate them since the markers are gene products, i.e., proteins. A brief description of the microarray experiment would be included in a submission as background to describe the thought process on the choice of genes to follow up in the development of the mechanistic hypothesis. Submission of the gene expression data in this example would be limited to the effect of the compound on the Notch pathway. The definitive supporting evidence for the safety claim would be provided by data from experiments assessing the activity of the protein biomarkers.

A Hypothetical Submission in Support of the Safety Claims for a Hypolipidemic Drug

An example based on a hypolipidemic drug of the PPARα agonist class is a good case where toxicity (liver cancer) is found in rodents and there is a good understanding documented in the literature of how this toxicity should not be a concern for humans under conditions of normal therapeutic use [4]. Furthermore, many laboratories have microarray data available from studies of these compounds with which to test the case and explore how much of these data would be required for regulatory purposes and assessment of potential human risk. A brief description of this example is shown in Box 11.2.

For this PPARα agonist, as for the gamma secretase example, it may be sufficient to show the statistically significant (and processed) data with emphasis on those pieces of data used to make the case for safety, with reference to published data. This may be a case where the sponsor is using an in-house experiential database for reference. One question is how much of that experiential data from reference compounds would need to be submitted in addition to data derived from the drug itself? The differentially expressed genes identified in the study were considered to be the same genes that have been well established as part of the cascade of transcriptional events elicited by activation of the PPARα [5]. Hence, this set of genes represents a drug safety biomarker, and the performance of this specific set of genes requires further validation. The latter may or may not involve the use of microarray technology but does not require whole genome expression data.

Highlights from the Discussions

The group found it difficult to come up with a case example where microarray data prove a hypothesis/mechanism. Rather, it was felt that toxicogenomics data help most in formulating hypotheses. When the science advances to a point where specific gene expression changes are widely accepted as qualified and fit for use in regulatory toxicological evaluations as known or probable valid biomarkers, then microarray data may become more frequently used for supporting hypotheses. The group proposed that such

---

BOX 11.2   CASE EXAMPLE 2: TOXICOGENOMIC ANALYSIS OF NOFATATOL IN RAT LIVER

BACKGROUND

Nofatatol is a hypothetical PPARα agonist indicated as adjunctive therapy to diet to reduce elevated LDL-C, Total C, Triglycerides and Apo B and to increase HDL-C in patients with hypercholesterolemia or mixed dyslipidemia. Pre-clinical development studies indicate that it is a non-genotoxic liver carcinogen in rodents. A global gene expression profiling approach using microarrays was undertaken to examine the gene expression changes induced in rat liver by Nofatatol. Such gene expression profiling has previously shown that fibric acid analogs that have been associated with hepatic tumors in rats induce hepatomegaly in this species through activation of the PPARα with subsequent peroxisome proliferation.

RESULTS

The gene expression results for Nofatatol were compared to those for Wy-14643 and for clofibrate (both PPARα agonists) as well as with data from a reference database of other liver carcinogens. Predictive modeling algorithms indicated that Nofatatol has a high potential for causing: enzyme induction and liver enlargement; peroxisome proliferation; and liver tumors by a non-genotoxic mechanism. Furthermore, compound similarity calculations showed a high correlation between Nofatatol and peroxisome proliferators including Wy-14643 and clofibrate. The results strongly suggest that Nofatatol acts via the PPARα mediated pathway, inducing genes in rodents which are not induced in humans [6,7]. The toxicogenomic analysis clearly identified Nofatatol as one of the class of compounds activating PPARα and inducing peroxisome proliferation in rat liver. The latter activity has been associated with the induction of liver tumors in rodents, by mechanisms that are not re-capitulated in humans, hence should not be considered to be relevant to human risk [4,6,7].

---

data mostly provide a starting point for the identification of more definitive biomarkers that will need further qualification studies for acceptance. The major questions and comments raised can be summarized as follows.

Can the Type of Data be Categorized in Order to Pose Appropriate Questions?

Yes, data may be generated:

- From early discovery exploratory profiling
- For hypothesis generation to explain a pre-clinical finding
- For hypothesis generation to explain a clinical finding
- As biomarkers of safety/efficacy
- For hypothesis confirmation supporting risk/benefit assessment

How May the Examples be Categorized?

- The gamma-secretase example initially fits the 'pre-clinical hypothesis generation' category although it is based on an understanding of the pharmacology of the drug.

The gene expression data provide support for a hypothesis that is later confirmed and is based on the drug affecting the Notch pathway. Another outcome from the gene expression experiments in this example is the identification of a biomarker for the gastrointestinal damage which can be monitored in the clinic.

- The PPAR alpha agonist example fits the 'hypothesis confirmation' category if the sponsor and reviewer agree that the gene expression changes are known to be associated with this class of compound and indicative of a rodent-specific mechanism of hepatocarcinogenesis.

From a Regulatory Perspective, How Much Data Do Reviewers Want to See and How Much Data Must a Sponsor Provide? Should Submissions include All the Data Up Front or Only Those Known or Probable Valid Data Elements Relevant to the Arguments Made in the Assessment by the Sponsor?

1. The reviewer should have sufficient data to make a 'knowledgeable judgment'; that is, to either confirm or refute the sponsor's arguments. The full data sets may be made available at the request of the reviewer, if needed.

How Should Data be Presented?

2. The group came to the consensus that the data should be presented:
- Concentrating on a subset of the statistically significant changes in gene expression.
- To show the results for all known and probable valid biomarkers that have been commonly established prior to the time of submission.
- To show the data that were selected by the sponsor for further qualification/validation to address the arguments/interpretations being made by the sponsor (with details of the rationale for how the selection was made). These new endpoints are essentially being proposed by the sponsor to be qualified as new probable valid biomarkers of the toxicity.
- Optionally and voluntarily with a summary table of those changes in gene expression not used in developing the safety claim. Explanation of such changes may not be necessary unless there is a clear signal relevant to drug safety. Interpretation in context, i.e., with reference to all findings in the study, is important.

What Depth of Data Needs to be Submitted?

3. For the PPAR agonist and the gamma secretase examples, it may be sufficient to show the statistically significant (and processed) data with emphasis on those pieces of data used to make the case for safety, with reference to published data.
4. There may be cases where the sponsor is using an in-house experiential database. A question is how much of the experiential data would need to be submitted?

How Much Data are Enough (How Raw, How Much Proof of Reliability, How Much Detail on Process)?

5. Details of the processing of the data are very important in this respect to ensure that a reviewer can critically evaluate how a sponsor has arrived at interpretations.
6. The group can build recommendations using the example cases.
7. The gamma secretase example includes the identification of a safety biomarker.
   - In this case the gene expression data, although needed to identify the marker, are not needed to validate it.
   - The validation is done independently of the gene expression study.
   - Submission of the gene expression data would focus on the effect of the compound on the Notch pathway in this example.

What are the Main Statistical Considerations?

8. Statistical outcomes are dependent on the quality of the array data. The group highlighted the need to get a sense of mutually accepted criteria for quality assurance (QA) and analysis.
9. A comparison in ArrayTrack of two different statistical approaches yielded c.100 gene expression changes by either approach, but there was only a 50% overlap of the genes identified. However, each gene set gave the same biological interpretation when pathways were used in the analysis.

What About Microarray Data Obtained from Efficacy Studies?

10. In addition to providing supportive evidence for efficacy, data from discovery studies may yield interpretations suggesting the potential for a toxic effect associated with certain classes of agent, since toxicity is often a result of exaggerated pharmacological effects.
11. A good safety claim may be made for a compound based on the lack of any observed pathology but these additional data may raise some safety concerns.
12. However, the safety concerns may be monitorable in the clinic and could be tested in longer term pre-clinical studies, provided they are not life-threatening or irreversible.
13. A big question is to the extent to which data from an efficacy study should be used to support a case for safety.
14. Would the data be interpreted by a discovery team and not seen by a safety assessment representative?
15. Would a regulatory reviewer look for safety evaluation signals in the data (if there is an indication of drug-induced toxicity due to exaggerated pharmacologic effects)?
16. Since Code of Federal Regulations (CFR) requirements focus on submission of animal toxicity data that are specifically generated in Good Laboratory Practice

(GLP) studies to support the safety of clinical testing, then the decision to include efficacy data of this kind is likely to be with the sponsor. There is no regulatory mandate to provide data from non-GLP animal efficacy studies used for internal business decision making, and not for supporting the safe conduct of clinical trials.

17. Data from studies in efficacy models are not always taken into account in the safety assessment by some review divisions (e.g., oncology drugs), but are considered important in others.

18. From the perspective of data standards, the submission of data from efficacy studies could follow the same template as proposed for toxicogenomic submissions.

19. As for toxicogenomic studies, the microarray approach may be used to identify small sets of genes that would then be followed up by studies using qRT-PCR or enzyme-linked immunosorbent assay (ELISA) (for gene product). In such a case it may not be necessary to submit these preliminary microarray data.

20. The data may be appropriate for a Voluntary Exploratory Data Submission (VXDS) in which case raw data are preferred to enable training of reviewers to see how microarray data are analyzed. N.B.: There is no obligation to submit to VXDS and there are no absolute requirements for submission format. VXDS data will not be used for regulatory decisions.

Conclusions

The final document produced by the team with its recommendations can be obtained on request from info@discotox.co.uk.

The approach taken by this group proved to be an excellent way for debating the issues of standards in toxicogenomic submissions. Working backwards from the submission phase of the mock case examples, and forward through the steps leading from experimental design through data generation and interpretation, helped the team to identify key components for data submission standards. The gene expression experiments for these examples would have benefited from a targeted gene approach, which would have improved the statistical analysis framework for these data compared to that for data of whole genome microarrays.

The team felt the emphasis should be on simplicity and relevance in presenting to the regulatory agencies the major findings of toxicogenomic data, as well as clarity in describing the analytical methods used to process the data and the thought process leading to the conclusions of the sponsor. At least some discussants thought it important not to over-interpret toxicogenomic data, and that their context relevant to other toxicological findings was important, particularly if the toxicogenomic findings were from exploratory studies. The draft submission template presents a guide to what pieces of information should be made available, and in what format, by the sponsor for the regulatory agency to make a critical and independent review. A reviewer should be able to request more extensive data submission (i.e., all the raw, unprocessed data) on a case by case basis. It is of benefit to both sponsor and reviewer to follow current agreed data standards and published guidance. The team did an excellent job in identifying the outstanding issues and especially the philosophy by which standards should be applied.

Acknowledgments

I thank the following for their active participation in the discussion group described in this vignette. Gregory Akerman, Supratim Choudhuri, David Dix, Kellye Daniels, Feleke Eshete, Jennifer Fostel, Sabine Francke, Lois Freed, Felix Frueh, Jim Fuscoe, Federico Goodsaid, David Hattan, Kenneth Haymes, George Ikeda, Ying Jiang, Mike Lawton, John Leighton, Bill Mattes, Nancy McCarroll, Alex Nie, Mike Orr, Tom Papoian, Syril Pettit, Scott Pine, Susanna Sansone, George Searfoss, Ron Snyder, Frank Sistare, Joe Sina, Jim Stevens, Laura Suter-Dick, Scott Thurmond, Weida Tong, Roger Ulrich, Mike Waters.

References

[1] Pennie W, Pettit SD, Lord PG. Toxicogenomics in risk assessment: an overview of an HESI collaborative research program. Environ Health Perspect 2004;112:417–9.

[2] Searfoss GH, Jordan WH, Calligaro DO, Galbreath EJ, Schirtzinger LM, Berridge BR, et al. Adipsin, a biomarker of gastrointestinal toxicity mediated by a functional gamma-secretase inhibitor. J Biol Chem 2003;278:46107–16.

[3] Milano J, McKay J, Dagenais C, Foster-Brown L, Pognan F, Gadient R, et al. Modulation of notch processing by gamma-secretase inhibitors causes intestinal goblet cell metaplasia and induction of genes known to specify gut secretory lineage differentiation. Toxicol Sci 2004;82:341–58.

[4] Cattley RC, DeLuca J, Elcombe C, Fenner-Crisp P, Lake BG, Marsman DS, et al. Do peroxisome proliferating compounds pose a hepatocarcinogenic hazard to humans? Regul Toxicol Pharmacol 1998;27:47–60.

[5] Baker VA, Harries HM, Waring JF, Duggan CM, Ni HA, Jolly RA, et al. Clofibrate-induced gene expression changes in rat liver: a cross-laboratory analysis using membrane cDNA arrays. Environ Health Perspect 2004;12:428–38.

[6] Ammerschlaeger M, Beigel J, Klein KU, Mueller SO. Characterization of the species-specificity of peroxisome proliferators in rat and human hepatocytes. Toxicol Sci 2004;78:229–40.

[7] Lawrence JW, Li Y, Chen S, DeLuca JG, Berger JP, Umbenhauer DR, et al. Differential gene regulation in human versus rodent hepatocytes by peroxisome proliferator-activated receptor (PPAR) alpha. PPAR alpha fails to induce peroxisome proliferation-associated genes in human cells independently of the level of receptor expression. J Biol Chem 2001;276:31521–7.

12

Biomarker Qualification – Past, Present and Future

Initiating a Cross-Sector Toxicogenomics Biomarker Initiative – Health and Environmental Sciences Institute (HESI) Committee on Application of Genomics to Mechanism-Based Risk Assessment

Denise Robinson-Gravatt[1], Jiri Aubrecht[1], Raegan O'Lone[2], Syril Pettit[2]

[1]PFIZER INC., GROTON, CONNECTICUT, USA, [2]HESI, WASHINGTON DC, USA

Against the backdrop of the launch of the Human Genome Project, scientists from a variety of industries, academia and governmental organizations convened in late 1998 under the sponsorship of the International Life Sciences Institute (ILSI) Health and Environmental Sciences Institute (HESI) to deliberate on how best to advance the promising field of toxicogenomics. The landmark undertaking to sequence the human genome was enabled by the emergence of a variety of approaches and platforms for measuring changes in the expressions of thousands of genes simultaneously, and there was widespread interest in the toxicology community in applying this knowledge and the emerging technologies to safety assessment.

This chapter describes the role played by the HESI Committee on the Application of Genomics to Mechanism-based Risk Assessment (HESI Genomics Committee) in facilitating a cross-industry, government and academic effort to explore the utility of genomics methods and technologies for improving the understanding of mechanisms of toxicity and advancing risk assessment, and its contributions to the development of multi-site biomarker validation approaches. Since its establishment in 1999, the HESI Genomics Committee has evolved from evaluating a variety of gene array technologies, through performing pivotal proof of concept studies, to leading and supporting the application of toxicogenomics in risk assessment and regulatory decision making. The Committee's groundbreaking efforts in comparing platform performance and gene expression reproducibility across sites and applications has served as foundational work underlying many current biomarker qualification approaches.

The Path from Biomarker Discovery to Regulatory Qualification. http://dx.doi.org/10.1016/B978-0-12-391496-5.00012-0

HESI's Contributions to the Emerging Field of Toxicogenomics

In the late 1990s, the potential utility of genomic data for assessing compound-induced toxicity was a nascent field. The notion that detecting mRNA levels of multiple genes in parallel could offer a 'gene signature', providing more comprehensive information on underlying biologic processes, was enabled by the advent of newly developed gene 'array' technologies. Initial published studies [1–4] indicated that 'gene signatures' could be used for the differentiation of toxic from nontoxic substances, and toxicogenomics as a scientific discipline was born. Toxicogenomics, as any emerging field of science that employs a maturing technology, was challenged with issues of analytical sensitivity and reproducibility, cross-platform variability, multiple sources of sequence data, different and inconsistent approaches for data analysis, and a general lack of informatics capability.

The effort of the HESI Genomics Committee in its early years (1999–2005) focused on evaluation of analytical technologies and evaluation of the gene signature concept [2–5]. Given the novelty of the technology, the Committee recognized the importance of assessing potential sources of technical as well as biological variability and the value of a broad consortium effort to do so. The unique combination of academic, government, and industry laboratory scientists participating in the HESI Genomics Committee offered the opportunity for a multi-site and multi-sector approach to addressing the biological and technological questions at hand [6–10]. Only by pooling expertise as well as financial and laboratory resources was it possible to evaluate what was, at that point, a very time consuming and expensive methodological approach.

HESI established a baseline evaluation of the technical performance of the available microarray assay systems through a variety of endpoints. Experimental protocols were designed to assess the impact of variability in extraction and processing protocols, laboratory reagents, scanner settings, and data capture and analysis software [11–14]. To provide insights into the biology underlying highly investigated areas of compound-induced toxicity, the program assessed the potential for genomic microarrays to generate reproducible signatures of gene expression in the areas of hepatotoxicity, nephrotoxicity and genotoxicity. Three multi-sector working groups were formed to design studies in these areas [13,15,16]. There was consensus around the importance of anchoring changes in gene expression to recognized and well accepted toxicological and histopathologic endpoints. However, such anchoring posed some challenges, as the histopathologic manifestation of the toxic effects of chemicals is a product of changes arising over time. In contrast, toxicogenomic analyses provide a snapshot into the physiology of the cell at the moment that the RNA was isolated. From these early studies came important insights related to overall study design, which lead to recommendations that study protocols be optimized with respect to both gene expression endpoints as well as standard histopathology.

Although the HESI Genomics Committee's efforts provided positive steps forward, the process was challenged by the state of the science at the time. In the late 1990s and early

2000s, accessible gene annotations and bioinformatics analysis tools were very limited. As such, the observed gene expression signatures in these early studies were defined primarily by their statistical, not biological or molecular pathway, significance. The Committee recognized and reported on the need to develop and publish pathways to contextualize the changes in gene expression. Subsequent efforts to develop pathway analysis tools (that are so plentiful today) were likely influenced by the Committee's publicized recommendations in this regard. It is also worth noting that the Committee's early work related to genomic markers of nephrotoxicity laid the groundwork for further research by a number of investigators. These efforts culminated in extensive biomarker qualification work through HESI [5,13] and the Critical Path Institute's Predictive Safety Testing Consortium [17], with an initial set of renal safety biomarkers qualified in 2009 for use in studies intended to be submitted in support of new drug registrations.

The HESI Genomic Committee's early work also demonstrated that individual gene expression (via microarray) was challenging to reproduce, but that panels of associated genes relevant to specific pathways could be reliably reproduced across sites. This finding, while perhaps taken for granted in 2012, provided an important foundation for characterizing future biomarkers of effect and the degree of natural biological variations in gene expression. The Committee furthered this work in a 2006 meta-analysis of microarray data from untreated or vehicle-treated animals consisting of over 500 Affymetrix microarrays from control rat liver and kidney from 16 different institutions which identified gender, organ section, strain and fasting state as key sources of variability [10]. The most variable (gender-selective) and least variable (altered by fasting) contributors were also identified and functionally categorized [8,10]. This led to the identification of key descriptors which should be included in the minimal information about a toxicogenomics study to enable meaningful interpretation of results. Collectively, the Committee's work along with others in the field defined the need for the interpretation of toxicogenomic data in the context of molecular pathways and pathways-based biomarkers [18].

Use of Toxicogenomics to Biological Assess Mechanisms – Case Studies

Case Study on Application of Toxicogenomics to Elucidate Mechanisms of Genotoxicity

The Genotoxicity Working Group's initial objective was to evaluate the utility of gene expression profile analysis for risk assessment of genotoxicants. The group developed and analyzed gene expression profiles of compounds with known mechanisms of genotoxicity to determine whether compounds from different mechanistic classes displayed distinct gene expression profiles. The data from the initial round of studies supported the hypothesis that gene expression profiles could be used to discriminate between broad classes of genotoxicants (e.g., DNA-reactive genotoxicants from indirect/non-DNA-reactive genotoxicants)

[19,20]. The Committee has further validated these initial findings through more expansive sets of test compounds and implementation of a specific gene expression-optimized study protocol that was originally developed in Dr. Albert Fornace's laboratory at Georgetown University [21]. The resulting multi-laboratory studies coordinated by the Genotoxicity Working Group [12] have supported the potential for genomic biomarker signatures to be used as specific markers of genetic toxicity.

In order to demonstrate the applicability of the genomic biomarker approach for de-risking of irrelevant positive findings in the *in vitro* chromosome aberration assays, a Pfizer-sponsored Voluntary Genomics Data Submission (VXDS) was presented to the FDA (Food and Drugs Administration) with caffeine as a case study [18]. The feedback from the FDA on the scientific validity of the genomic biomarker approach and its potential application for regulatory risk assessment, including the agency support to advance a formal biomarker qualification program, was the major impetus for initiating the HESI Genomic Biomarker Qualification Project that is currently in progress. The goal of this project is to achieve regulatory qualification of the genomic biomarker approach for de-risking of positive findings in the *in vitro* chromosome damage assays as outlined in the VXDS. The studies to be submitted for qualification utilize a combined RT-PCR and microarray based approach to assess compounds in defined mechanistic classes. The study is anticipated to generate an expression signature (genomic biomarker) that will differentiate DNA from non-DNA-reactive mechanisms of genotoxicity. The qualification submission will also propose specific 'contexts of use' for these genomic biomarkers with regard to safety/risk decision making. Qualification of such a biomarker approach is anticipated to limit the need for additional *in vivo* testing and simplify genetic safety risk assessment for drugs and chemicals.

The HESI Genomics Committee has also partnered with scientists and organizations with similar interests in facilitating improved approaches to genotoxicity risk assessment. A collaboration was formed with the Europe-based carcinoGENOMICS consortium (http://www.carcinogenomics.eu/), European Center for Validation of Alternative Methods (http://ecvam.jrc.it/), and the Netherlands Genomics Initiative (http://www.genomics.nl/) which resulted in an international workshop 'Genomics in Cancer Risk Assessment' held in 2009 (all URLs accessed June 10, 2013). The workshop brought together scientists from academia, industry and regulatory agencies to discuss the development and application of a new genomic-based paradigm for the assessment of genetic safety and carcinogenicity. A 'road map' for this paradigm shift that includes products of the Genotoxicity Working Group and its genomic biomarker qualification efforts, as well as methods developed via the CarcinoGENOMICS consortium, is described in Paules et al. [22].

Case Study on the Application of Toxicogenomics to Elucidate Mechanisms of Cardiotoxicity

HESI's Mechanism-Based Markers of Toxicity (Doxorubicin Study) Working Group designed and implemented a six-week study in a rodent model of doxorubicin-induced cardiotoxicity to assess the power of genomic data to yield mechanistic insights into toxicity. The study assessed standard endpoints, such as histopathology, clinical chemistry and cardiac troponin in parallel with an extensive collection of microarray data. The study was designed to include a dose and time response, treatment with a compound that is pharmacologically similar to doxorubicin but does not cause cardiotoxicity, a group dosed with adjuvant therapy used clinically to reduce doxorubicin-associated toxicity, as well as recovery groups. These different treatment groups were included to evaluate the influence of study design, experimental methods, and data analysis approaches on toxicogenomic studies. The analysis of the study is ongoing, but interim results suggest that it will provide an in-depth example of the use of genomics as a means of enhancing the mechanistic understanding of compound toxicity, and will provide insight into the relationship between time, dose, gene expression and the onset of toxicity. The results of this extensive set of studies hold promise for identification of novel markers of doxorubicin-related toxicity. Furthermore, in expression profiling experiments for microRNAs upregulated in cardiac tissue derived from the doxorubicin treated samples of this study, several microRNAs were identified as induced by doxorubicin, and correlated to repression of mRNA targets in this same tissue [23]. Regulation of both microRNA and mRNA in advance of overt toxicity presents potential opportunities for biomarker development.

Current Focus and Activities of the HESI Genomics Committee

With the experience gained through their efforts evaluating technical issues, sources of variability, and data analysis approaches associated with the use of toxicogenomics in pre-clinical studies, HESI Genomics Committee projects continue to expand into practical applications of toxicogenomics for risk assessment, generating biomarker and other data of relevance for regulatory practice.

The discovery of circulating microRNA species in blood and their potential to be used as tissue specific biomarkers of drug-induced injury [24] has provided new and exciting opportunities for biomarker research. Similar to the state of transcriptomics (detecting levels of mRNA in tissues) in the late 1990s, there are a wide range of technologies and protocols emerging for detection of circulating microRNAs. Building on their historical experience in understanding and optimizing novel technology platforms, and based on the broad interest in microRNAs as biomarkers of injury, the HESI Genomics Committee designed a multi-laboratory study to evaluate best practices for assessment of microRNAs in biofluids for drug-induced injury. Employing a rodent model of isoproterenol-induced cardiac injury, multiple sites are analyzing blood and urine samples derived from a single in-life study for a uniform set of microRNA markers, utilizing a standard protocol and defined protocol modifications. From this study, a better understanding of the sources of variation in assessments of microRNAs is expected. Once complete, recommendations will be published for standard protocols for reliable and reproducible detection of microRNAs in biofluids. These standardized approaches could be employed across laboratories and thus facilitate the further development of microRNA data that can be queried toward identification of potential novel and improved biomarkers for toxicology studies.

In collaboration with Pfizer and the Hamner Institutes, the HESI Genomics Committee is furthering its efforts to define genomic mechanisms through the use of inbred mouse strains that model genetic diversity in the human population [25,26]. These studies incorporate traditional toxicology endpoints as well as transcriptomic profiling to assess variances in drug-induced responses in inbred mouse strains. The outcome of this program will ultimately provide perspective on the utility of these models for detecting drug-induced injury as well as elucidating biological mechanisms through a genomic assessment. By generating data on the role of genetic diversity in the presentation and detection of adverse responses in rodent models, this work will inform approaches to the translation of animal model data to clinical relevance.

Summary and Future Horizons

Over the past 15 years, toxicogenomics, as an approach based on transcriptomics, has evolved from a novel and technically challenging method into a technologically and scientifically feasible approach. The initial excitement about its potential to replace classical toxicologic and pathologic methods was overly optimistic and its major impact on regulatory decision making still remains to be realized. Nevertheless, toxicogenomic applications are now routinely used in many organizations to complement and inform mechanistic evaluations. The work of the HESI Genomics Committee significantly facilitated the scientific community's understanding of the potential as well as the limitations of the technology.

New project opportunities continue to present themselves to the toxicogenomics community as our understanding of biology evolves and new technologies emerge. The Genomics Committee is establishing plans for an analysis of formalin fixed paraffin embedded (FFPE) tissues to enable transcriptomic profiling via next generation sequencing of these generally inaccessible tissues due to RNA degradation. Technology allowing genomic analysis of FFPE tissues has been a long-standing need for toxicological and clinical research.

The Committee is assembling resources and expertise for generation of a microRNA expression atlas of the rat. This map is anticipated to facilitate microRNA research and to advance exploration of these microRNAs as potential biomarkers. A better understanding of the tissue distribution of microRNAs in untreated rat tissues will aid the interpretation of alterations of miRNA signatures and expression level changes that may occur upon drug or chemical treatment. Knowledge of baseline (untreated) expression levels will also assist in better interpreting microRNA expression changes in biofluids in response to disease or compound treatment, and will facilitate identification of promising new biomarkers of site-specific injury. Additionally, the conduct of this program on a next generation sequencing platform will allow for further evaluation of this technology as a means for detecting and assessing microRNA expression.

For over a decade, the HESI Genomics Committee has conducted successful, collaborative programs to evaluate technologies for genomics assessments, explore and establish standardization of methods, enhance data analysis and reporting, and share information with the scientific community based on pooled knowledge, resources, and expertise. With lessons learned from the initial technology evaluations, the Committee will now seek to facilitate genomic biomarker development with methods in more routine use (e.g., reverse transcription-polymerase chain reaction (RT-PCR) and microarrays) as well as more emergent technologies (next generation sequencing). These programs will contribute to the knowledge of fundamental biology and mechanism of action, as with the doxorubicin study and microRNA atlas, and add to the repertoire of assessments for toxicity evaluations.

References

[1] Waring JF, Jolly RA, Ciurlionis R, Lum PY, Praestgaard JT, Morfitt DC, et al. Clustering of hepatotoxins based on mechanism of toxicity using gene expression profiles. Toxicol Appl Pharmacol 2001;175:28–42.

[2] Hamadeh HK, Bushel PR, Jayadev S, Martin K, DiSorbo O, Sieber S, et al. Gene expression analysis reveals chemical-specific profiles. Toxicol Sci 2002;67:219–31.

[3] Hamadeh HK, Bushel P, Paules R, Afshari CA. Discovery in toxicology: mediation by gene expression array technology. J Biochem Mol Toxicol 2001;15:231–42.

[4] Hamadeh HK, Knight BL, Haugen AC, Sieber S, Amin RP, Bushel PR, et al. Methapyrilene toxicity: anchorage of pathologic observations to gene expression alterations. Toxicol Pathol 2002;30:470–82.

[5] Pennie W, Pettit SD, Lord PG. Toxicogenomics in risk assessment: an overview of an HESI collaborative research program. Environ Health Perspect 2004;112:417–9.

[6] Goodsaid FM, Smith RJ, Rosenblum IY. Quantitative PCR deconstruction of discrepancies between results reported by different hybridization platforms. Environ Health Perspect 2004;112:456–60.

[7] Mattes WB, Pettit SD, Sansone SA, Bushel PR, Waters MD. Database development in toxicogenomics: issues and efforts. Environ Health Perspect 2004;112:495–505.

[8] Corton JC, Bushel PR, Fostel J, O'Lone RB. Sources of variance in baseline gene expression in the rodent liver. Mutat Res 2012;746(2):104–12.

[9] Rosenzweig BA, Pine PS, Domon OE, Morris SM, Chen JJ, Sistare FD. Dye bias correction in dual-labeled cDNA microarray gene expression measurements. Environ Health Perspect 2004;112:480–7.

[10] Boedigeimer MJ, Wolfinger RD, Bass MB, Bushel PR, Chou JW, Cooper M, et al. Sources of variation in baseline gene expression levels from toxicogenomics study control animals across multiple laboratories. BMC Genomics 2008;9:285.

[11] Baker VA, Harries HM, Waring JF, Duggan CM, Ni HA, Jolly RA, et al. Clofibrate-induced gene expression changes in rat liver: a cross-laboratory analysis using membrane cDNA arrays. Environ Health Perspect 2004;112:428–38.

[12] Ellinger-Ziegelbauer H, Fostel JM, Aruga C, Bauer D, Boitier E, Deng S, et al. Characterization and interlaboratory comparison of a gene expression signature for differentiating genotoxic mechanisms. Toxicol Sci 2009;110:341–52.

[13] Ulrich RG, Rockett JC, Gibson GG, Pettit SD. Overview of an interlaboratory collaboration on evaluating the effects of model hepatotoxicants on hepatic gene expression. Environ Health Perspect 2004;112:423–7.

[14] Waring JF, Ulrich RG, Flint N, Morfitt D, Kalkuhl A, Staedtler F, et al. Interlaboratory evaluation of rat hepatic gene expression changes induced by methapyrilene. Environ Health Perspect 2004;112: 439–48.

[15] Amin RP, Vickers AE, Sistare F, Thompson KL, Roman RJ, Lawton M, et al. Identification of putative gene based markers of renal toxicity. Environ Health Perspect 2004;112:465–79.

[16] Newton RK, Aardema M, Aubrecht J. The utility of DNA microarrays for characterizing genotoxicity. Environ Health Perspect 2004;112:420–2.

[17] Dieterle F, Sistare F, Goodsaid F, Papaluca M, Ozer J, Webb C, et al. Renal biomarker qualification submission: a dialog between the FDA-EMA and Predictive Safety Testing Consortium. Nature Biotech 2010;28(5):455–62.

[18] Goodsaid FM, Amur S, Aubrecht J, Burczynski ME, Carl K, Catalano J, et al. Voluntary exploratory data submissions to the US FDA and the EMA: experience and impact. Nat Rev Drug Discov 2010;9: 435–45.

[19] Newton RK, Aardema M, Aubrecht JA. Environ Health Persp 2004;112(4):420–2.

[20] Dickinson DA, Warnes GR, Quievryn G, Messer J, Zhitkovich A, Rubitski E, et al. Differentiation of DNA reactive and non-reactive genotoxic mechanisms using gene expression profile analysis. Mutat Res 2004;18(1–2):29–41. 549.

[21] Amundson SA, Do KT, Vinikoor L, Koch-Paiz CA, Bittner ML, Trent JM, et al. Stress-specific signatures: expression profiling of p53 wild-type and -null human cells. Oncogene 2005;30(28): 4572–9. 24.

[22] Paules RS, Aubrecht J, Corvi R, Garthoff B, Kleinjans JC. Moving forward in human cancer risk assessment. Environ Health Perspect 2011;119(6):739–43.

[23] Vacchi-Suzzi C, Bauer Y, Berridge BR, Bonglovanni S, Gerrish K, Hamadeh HK, et al. Perturbation of microRNAs in rat heart during chronic doxorubicin treatment. PLOSone 2012;7(7):e40395. http://dx.doi.org/10.1371/journal.pone.0040395.

[24] Wang K, Zhang S, Marzolf B, Troisch P, Brightman A, Hu Z, et al. Proc Natl Acad Sci U S A 2009; 106(11):4402–7. Epub 2009 Feb 25.

[25] Harrill AH, Watkins PB, Su S, Ross PK, Harbort DE, Stylianou IM, et al. Mouse population-guided resequencing reveals that variants in CD44 contribute to acetaminophen-induced liver injury in humans. Genome Res 2009;19(9):1507–15. Epub 2009 May 5.

[26] Liu HH, Lu P, Guo Y, Farrell E, Zhang X, Zheng M, et al. An integrative genomic analysis identifies Bhmt2 as a diet-dependent genetic factor protecting against acetaminophen-induced liver toxicity. Genome Res 2010;20(1):28–35.

SECTION

4

Biomarkers of Drug Safety

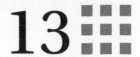

13

'Classic' Biomarkers of Liver Injury

John R. Senior

ASSOCIATE DIRECTOR FOR SCIENCE, FOOD AND DRUG ADMINISTRATION (FDA), SILVER SPRING, MARYLAND, USA

In the current frenzy to find new biomarkers (a search of the National Library of Medicine program PubMed in June 2013, for the entry biomarkers, yields over 600,000 published papers, increasing at more than 40,000 per year). It may be instructive to consider how a small set of serum chemical tests for liver injury or dysfunction came to be considered 'classic'. What are they and how did they come to deserve to be referred to as 'classic'? They are:

- serum concentration of total bilirubin (TBL),
- serum activity of alkaline phosphatase (ALP),
- serum activity of aspartate aminotransferase (AST), and
- serum activity of alanine aminotransferase (ALT).

Were they qualified, validated, or approved for use by methods described elsewhere in this book? Do they need to be in retrospect? My answer is 'no' and 'no'. Let us see why.

Bilirubin

In 1913, now almost a century ago, the Dutch physician Hijmans van den Bergh[a] and his young colleague Isadore Snapper, working in Groningen, The Netherlands, published an account [1] of a new method for distinguishing between jaundice caused by biliary obstruction and that from the rapid hemolysis of red blood cells, depending on whether the serum reacted immediately and 'directly' with an added reagent, or the reaction was

---

[a]Albert Abraham Hijmans van den Bergh was born in Rotterdam 1 December 1869, the son of Benjamin Hijmans and Berdina van den Bergh. The name Hijmans van den Bergh was therefore composed of both parents' surnames, although he is now referred to principally as van den Bergh. In Groningen, he and Isadore Snapper, a recent medical graduate, reported their findings in 1913 on the differences between direct and delayed-reacting bilirubin. Van den Bergh died 28 September 1943 in Utrecht, while fleeing and hiding from Gestapo pursuers [2]. Snapper had emigrated in 1938 to Brooklyn NY, then practiced at Mt. Sinai Hospital in New York City, where Hans Popper said he was a master of bedside medicine, a "physician for whom the word 'charisma' might have been invented".

The Path from Biomarker Discovery to Regulatory Qualification. http://dx.doi.org/10.1016/B978-0-12-391496-5.00013-2

'delayed' after ethanol was added. The reagent was aqueous sulfanilic-hydrochloric acid solution with a little freshly added sodium nitrite:

sulfanilic acid, 5 mg   sodium nitrite, 1.25 mg   Ehrlich diazo reagent

REACTION SCHEME 1

This gave a blue-violet color rapidly within 10–30 s if obstruction of the biliary system was present, but a slower development of reddish color deepening into violet in up to 15 min or more after the addition of alcohol, if hemolysis had occurred. The basis of the test was earlier work [3] by the German chemist Paul Ehrlich[b], who had found that a 'diazo reaction' occurred if bilirubin dissolved in chloroform or alcohol reacted with diazonium salts, such as the sulfanilic acid-nitrite reagent. Van den Bergh later found the reaction to be specific for the detection of bilirubin.

■ ■ ■ ▬▬▬▬▬▬▬▬▬▬▬▬▬▬▬▬▬▬▬▬▬▬▬▬▬▬▬▬▬▬▬▬▬▬▬▬▬

→ (This was indeed a biomarker, but the term was not to be invented for many decades!)

▬▬▬▬▬▬▬▬▬▬▬▬▬▬▬▬▬▬▬▬▬▬▬▬▬▬▬▬▬▬▬▬▬▬▬▬▬ ■ ■ ■

Scores of papers followed, many modifications were made, and better understanding gradually developed, but the work was confirmed over and over again for decades and millions of tests have been done. The original van den Bergh test was qualitative, but was clinically useful. Development of the photoelectric colorimeter in 1937 led to a test being produced by Helga Malloy and Kenneth Evelyn working at McGill University in Montreal. They measured [4] absorption by azobilirubin solutions of light transmitted by a filter at 540 μm to quantify both direct and total bilirubin (TBL) (the indirect bilirubin was the difference between total and direct bilirubin). By using diluted serum and absolute methanol, measurement of bilirubin became quantitative.

R. J. Cremer, a pediatric registrar in Essex, UK, discovered [5] in 1957 that bilirubin was light-sensitive by noting that serum bilirubin content decreased on serial observations of a sample exposed to light. Later, this observation became the basis for the phototherapy of newborn infants with hyperbilirubinemia (deficient clearance of plasma bilirubin formed from the physiologic hemolysis of fetal hemoglobin). The treatment prevented the neurotoxic effects of unconjugated bilirubin entering the brain.

[b]Paul Ehrlich (1854–1915), a brilliant German pathologist who was much interested in dyes and their reactions with cell and tissue receptors, had reported in Berlin in 1883 that a diazo reagent sulfanilic acid-acidic nitrite reacted with urinary pigments from jaundiced patients to produce a red-violet color. He developed arsphenamine (Salvorsan) as an anti-syphilitic agent, and received the Nobel Prize in Medicine for Physiology in 1908.

Dozens more slight modifications of testing methods were published, but the work of Rudi Schmid at the National Institute of Arthritis and Metabolic Diseases in Bethesda showed in 1956 that the direct-reacting bilirubin was a glucuronide conjugate [6], perhaps an ether at the α, α' hydroxyl groups, a more water-soluble compound than the unconjugated bilirubin that gave the delayed, indirect reaction. This work was concurrent with the report [7] by Billing and Lathe that the soluble forms of bilirubin were ester mono- and diglucuronides, at the propionic acid side-chains of the two middle pyrroles of bilirubin. Independently, Talafant from Brno in Czechoslovakia also reported [8] in the same year that the directly-reacting pigment was a glucuronide that could be split by bacterial or splenic β-glucuronidase, favoring an ester linkage. These insights then led rapidly to the elucidation by Arias and London [9] of the origin of the mild constitutional hyperbilirubinemia of Gilbert's syndrome [10] – a hepatic deficiency in a microsomal enzyme, UDPGT (uridine diphospho-glucuronyl transferase).

It became evident that the basis of the difference between directly and indirectly reacting bilirubin observed by van den Bergh was explained by the great differences in the water solubility of glucuronide-conjugated and unconjugated bilirubin. In plasma, almost all of the latter was bound to albumin [11]. Further work revealed the structure of bilirubin, and its origin in heme, the red pigment of the oxygen-carrying protein hemoglobin of red blood cells, with less heme coming from myoglobin, peroxidases, and cytochromes. In 1968, Schmid et al. at the University of California in San Francisco reported [12] that the cyclic tetrapyrrole of heme could be oxidized at the α-methanyl group by oxygen and NADPH, yielding a green pigment biliverdin, a linear tetrapyrrole, along with free iron, carbon monoxide, and NADP+ (nicotine adenine dinucleotide phosphate). The reaction was catalyzed by heme oxygenase, an enzyme he found in the liver, but which was 10 to 20 times more concentrated in splenic tissue, where most of the aged or damaged red blood cells were broken down. In the liver, heme oxygenase activity was associated with particulate fractions obtained by centrifugation of tissue homgenates to obtain the small particles of intracellular membranes called 'microsomes', in spleen and kidney homogenates.

REACTION SCHEME 2

The next step was conversion of green biliverdin to the yellow pigment bilirubin by another enzyme, biliverdin reductase [13], using NADH (nicotinamide dinucleotide) as a reducing agent. Originally studied in the liver, it was later purified also from the spleen, and found in other tissues.

REACTION SCHEME 3

The reaction between the Ehrlich reagent and bilirubin was then found [14] to result in two isomeric, dipyrrolic azopigments and formaldehyde from the central methylene carbon atom:

REACTION SCHEME 4

Another step in the story was the discovery [15,16] in Zurich of yet one more form of serum bilirubin, that of the so-called delta-bilirubin. This fourth type of bilirubin was later shown to be direct-reacting, covalently albumin-bound, and present in the plasma of patients with prolonged jaundice due to the impaired hepatic excretion of conjugated bilirubin [17].

As has been noted, free bilirubin was found to be poorly soluble in water and transported in plasma to liver bound to albumin by van der Waals forces. After transfer into the hepatocytes via intracellular binding proteins [18], the bilirubin is conjugated to mono- and diglucuronide esters, greatly increasing its water solubility for excretion into bile. Much continued to be learned about the several forms of bilirubin, internal hydrogen binding [19] of the unconjugated form, and powerful antioxidant properties [20] that continue to be investigated up to the present for possible use in the treatment of autoimmune disorders.

Alkaline phosphatase

We now know that the ALPs constitute a large number of zinc-metallo-protein enzymes that catalyze the hydrolytic breakdown of many organic phosphate compounds, that they are found in a very broad array of tissues, including bone, intestine, liver, placenta, and that they exist in many variant isozyme forms. The application as a new method for diagnosing liver disease began in 1930 with the observation [21] by Morrell Roberts that two of his patients with obstructive liver disease showed greater elevations of blood ALP activity than one with 'catarrhal jaundice'. This was followed up in 1933 with a much more definitive work [22] that showed that 21 patients with a broad variety of problems with obstruction of the bile ducts had significantly greater blood ALP activities than 19 with toxic or catarrhal jaundice, with no overlap. In the original work, Roberts used a very simple substrate, β-glycerophosphate or glyceryl-2-phosphate, and measured the rate of release of free phosphate over time at pH 8.9, detecting the phosphate with molybdic acid and hydroquinone to develop a blue color. Aaron Bodansky, working at the Hospital for Joint Diseases in New York, reported improvements in the accuracy of serum phosphate determination [23], and shortly afterwards, Earl King and Riley Armstrong from the Banting Institute in Toronto reported [24] that using phenylphosphate as substrate of the phosphatase reaction gave even better results.

REACTION SCHEME 5

They expressed the measurements of enzymatic ALP activity as mg of product produced per unit time under the conditions specified by the investigators. Thus began a long series of test improvements in both the substrates used and methods to detect products that has confused readers to this day, as the measurement of serum alkaline phosphatase activity (ALP) is still not entirely standardized. For example, Bodansky units for ALP are based on mg P, and King-Armstrong units on mg phenol released; on a molar basis the latter are about three times those of the former, using molecular weights of phenol as 94.1 and P as 31.0, which became increasingly important as automated machines [25] were being developed for rapidly processing hundreds of serum samples in routine monitoring.

Attempts to bring order out of confusing terminology, i.e., the same enzymes referred to by several names, led in 1956 to establishment by the International Union of Biochemistry of an International Commission on Enzymes to tackle problems of classification and nomenclature [26].

That report established six major classes of enzymes:
1) oxidoreductases,
2) transferases,
3) hydrolases,
4) lyases,
5) isomerases,
6) ligases.

A standard name was assigned to each enzyme using a code beginning with EC, then a number for the main class, a second number for subclass, a third number for sub-subclass, and a fourth for the serial number of the enzyme, the numbers being separated by periods. Thus it was established that ALP was one of a family of phosphoric monoester hydrolases (EC 3.1.3), and ALP became EC 3.1.3.1. Methods for determining and reporting its activity were not standardized, however, so caution is still needed when interpreting results obtained by laboratories using various substrates, methods, conditions, and machines.

Although ALP had been used as an aid to the diagnosis of obstructive jaundice since the work of Roberts in 1930, there was no agreement on whether elevations were caused by a reduced ability of the liver to clear enzyme produced in bone or elsewhere, or by stimulated production of the enzyme in the liver. Studies done in the gastrointestinal research laboratory of Darwin Prockop [27], working at the Philadelphia General Hospital in the laboratory adjacent to mine (when we were working on the problem of post-tranfusion acute hepatitis [28]), provided some early answers. To avoid any contribution of bone or other tissues, they studied isolated cat liver perfused with the animal's own oxygenated blood for six hours. After collection of steady-state samples for measuring ALP by a modified Bodansky method, the bile flow was measured hourly in three of seven cats, and in the other four the bile ducts were ligated. No elevation of serum ALP was noted in the animals with free flow of bile, but those with bile duct occlusion showed 4.5-fold rises in ALP levels. Assay of liver homogenates confirmed the rise in liver tissue ALP activities in animals with bile duct occlusion.

The findings of Prockop and his group were consistent with those of Polin et al. [29], and were confirmed by Marshall Kaplan [30] and colleagues about the same time as by workers in Germany [31]. Nevertheless, attempts at standardization by declaration did not resolve the bickering [32, 33]. Of more pertinent interest, early work [34] led to better instrumentation and equipment that allowed more precise localization of the liver ALP to the surfaces of hepatocytes [35], membranes [36], and especially of the canals of Hering and small bile ductules [37] but not the larger bile ducts. Over the 60 or so years of investigations into alkaline phosphatase as a serum biomarker of clinical usefulness, it became generally accepted as a cholestasis indicator, distinguishing between hepatocellular and cholestatic liver injury or disease [38]. In discussions in France over criteria for diagnosing drug-induced liver disorders as distinguished from those caused by disease, it was the consensus that the level of ALP, expressed as multiples of the upper limit of the normal range ($\times$ULN), relative to levels of enzyme activity markers of hepatocellular injury such as alanine aminotransferase (ALT) similarly expressed, could be used at the time of recognition of liver injury to define a ratio, R, that indicated a cholestatic process if ALT×ULN / ALP×ULN was < 2, primarily hepatocellular injury if > 5, and mixed, if in between.

Alternative and Discarded Biomarkers

As studies of bilirubin and alkaline phophatase were proceeding, other biomarkers were proposed and used to some extent, including the cephalin flocculation and thymol turbidity tests. In 1939, Franklin Hanger of New York described a new test for disturbances of the hepatic parenchyma based on the capacity of serum from patients with jaundice to floc-culate a colloidal suspension of cholesterol-cephalin complex derived from sheep brain. He had reported this to the Association of American Physicians in 1938 as a preliminary finding, but published a definitive paper [39] in the *Journal of Clinical Investigation* the next year. The test result were graded as + to ++++, and he claimed that no flocculation occurred with serum from patients with obstructive jaundice nor from normal human serum. His findings were not fully confirmed [40] by studies done by Pohle and Stewart in Madison WI, but they found it of some value in following the course of illness over time in patients with acute or sub-acute hepatitis. In later reports, Hanger and associates attempted to explain [41] the mechanism of the cephalin flocculation test as insufficiency of serum albumin to balance effects of increased gamma-globulin, or increased globulin to albumin ratio.

Another test, thymol turbidity, which appeared to be based on abnormal globulin released into plasma by diseased livers, was described [42] in 1944 by N. F. Maclagen, a biochemist at Westminster Hospital in Middlesex, UK. As an aid in the diagnosis of liver disease, it was realized that it was not a measure of any function of the liver but instead indicated dysfunction [43]. The test was done by adding serum from patients to barbital buffer saturated with thymol, showing turbidity if sera from patients with acute and chronic hepatitis. In a follow-up study of patients with disorders that were not primarily hepatic (malaria, rheumatoid arthritis, heart failure, glandular fever, sub-acute bacterial endocarditis) but in whom liver involvement was reported, mixed results [44] were obtained by Maclagen's laboratory. The cephalin flocculation and thymol turbidity tests were used by clinicians in the 1940s and 1950s but were not found to provide reliable and useful clinical information. There were superseded by better tests in the mid-1950s, faded from the scene, and are unknown to medical house officers of recent generations.

Other tests have been proposed but have not been adopted for widespread clinical use, in some cases because they were redundant, but mainly because of insufficient specificity, giving false positive results in patients without the disorder being sought for diagnosis, particularly unreliable when the disorder was of rare incidence or prevalence so that the diagnostic value of a positive result was very low indeed. Among the alternative tests [45] still used by some physicians are serum enzymes γ-glutamyltransferase, lactate dehydroge-nase, isocitric dehydrogenase, 5'-nucleotidase, leucine aminopeptidase, glutathione-sulfotransferase, cholinesterase, glutamate dehydogenase and others. Also studied by some are concentrations of bile acids, serum albumin and various globulins. Another different category of tests includes measurements of the clearance of injected dyes such as bromsulfophthalein and indocyanine green, galactose clearance, synthesis rate of urea, oxidative metabolism of various substrates and collection of expired radioactive or isotopic carbon dioxide. In general, these tests are not much used today because many of them are insensitive, unspecific, or cumbersome, time-consuming, laborious, and expensive [46].

Some of these have been proposed [47] as 'new' biomarkers, that might be more specific and perhaps even more sensitive than alanine aminotransferase, namely para-oxonase; malate, sorbitol, or glutamate dehydrogenase; and purine nucleoside phosphorylase, as readily measured by photometric methods and commercially available. Considered as costly were serum F protein, arginase I, and glutathione-sulfotransferase-α. We shall consider these proposals after looking at the development of the tests and methods for measuring activities of serum aspartate and alanine aminotransferase.

Aminotransferases (Transaminases)

In January 1955 a short added note in addendum [48] to another paper [49] was reported by a then recent medical graduate from New York University, containing findings that revolutionized the detection of acute liver disease and injury. Arthur Karmen[c] as a medical student helped two cardiologists to find new diagnostic biomarkers to diagnose acute myocardial infarction, by this reaction:

AST, aspartate aminotransferase
PALPO, pyridoxal phosphate
MDH, malic dehydrogenase
NADH, nicotine adenine dinucleotide

REACTION SCHEME 6

[c]Arthur Karmen, born 25 February 1930 in New York, was a medical student at New York University 1950–4. He worked with two cardiologists as mentors (John LaDue, Felix Wrobleski) on a search for new diagnostic biomarkers for acute myocardial infarction. He also worked with Severo Ochoa (1905–1993) who in 1936 had fled the civil war in Spain, wandered in Germany, England, and then to the United States and New York University in 1942, rising to become professor of biochemistry there in 1954. Ochoa shared the 1959 Nobel Prize in Physiology or Medicine with Arthur Kornberg, for their discoveries of ribonucleic acid (RNA) and deoxyribonucleic acid (DNA).

This reaction was the basis for the report, but the great advance was in the determination by spectrophotometric measurement at ultraviolet wavelength 340 μm of the disappearance of the reducing cofactor NADH (nicotine adenine dinucleotide) called at that time DPNH (diphospho-pyridine nucleotide, reduced). This made the test result rapidly reportable, with results in a few minutes instead of days, and suitable for automation in diagnostic testing machines.

It had been noted, even with the slow, cumbersome chromatographic assay of the glutamate produced, that addition of malic dehydrogenase to remove by catalyzed reduction the oxalacetate produced to malate, would make the main transamination reaction proceed smoothly.

Another enzyme found in heart and skeletal muscle, but at higher levels in liver tissue, was the serum glutamic-pyruvic transaminase (SGPT), which catalyzed the transfer of the amino group from alanine to α-ketoglutarate, giving rise to the later name of alanine aminotransferase (ALT, or ALAT). That reaction was also 'pulled' to the right by adding lactate dehydrogenase to speed the reduction of NADH, and spectrophotometric measurement at wavelength 340 mm.

ALT, alanine aminotransferase
PALPO, pyridoxal phosphate
LDH, lactate dehydrogenase
NADH, nicotine adenine dinucleotide

REACTION SCHEME 7

The genius of Arthur Karmen was realized in his many subsequent innovations in biochemical instrumentation, but none perhaps was of greater impact than the method for the rapid, automated assay of serum aminotransferase activities.[d] As a result of the Enzyme Commission's advice on nomenclature the enzymes were renamed for their substrates rather than their products, so SGOT became AST (or ASAT), EC 2.6.1.1, and SGPT became ALT (or ALAT), EC 2.6.1.2 in the new and current terminology.

---

[d]The findings of Karmen were so compelling that the author of this chapter, when he was an intern on the medical wards of the Hospital of the University of Pennsylvania in Philadelphia, obtained permission from the director of the hospital laboratory to use its equipment and facilities at night, when only emergency staff were on duty, to carry out measurements of serum transminase activities in patients, and performed hundreds of tests over the next year until the hospital laboratory was persuaded to take over the task.

As noted above, the discovery of the transaminase assays came out of the search for new biomarkers of myocardial infarction, initiated by cardiologists LaDue and Wroblewski, who in 1952 were studying post-operative myocardial infarction [50], and enlisted then-medical student Karmen in their efforts to search for a new method to detect cardiac injury. Their findings were first announced in September 1954, in a paper [51] describing use of the SGOT method to distinguish myocardial infarction in 16 patients from 22 with other cardiovascular diseases, 17 patients with neoplastic diseases, 14 with various infections, and 50 normal controls. The full paper, published in January 1955, provided details of the long, tedious chromatographic method for measuring the amount of glutamate produced by the transamination reaction, and the brief addendum note by Karmen detailing the new and very rapid spectrophotometric method. Wroblewski and LaDue also quickly recognized [52] the value of the method for assaying liver cell injury, but never thereafter worked with Karmen, who had left New York University to intern at Bellevue Hospital and then went to NIH to work on instrumentation.

The novel, simple, and cheap method for determining the activity of serum enzymes such as AST and ALT transformed clinical chemistry, and led to abandoning of poorly understood and unspecific cephalin flocculation and thymol turbidity tests in the late 1950s and early 1960s. Other methods for measuring serum aminotransferase activity using colorimetric methods based on the reaction of dinitrophenylhydrazine with pyruvate were described shortly afterwards by Reitman and Frankel [53]. In 1955 in Naples, Fernando De Ritis and colleagues described in the Italian literature their findings of increased serum transaminases in human epidemic viral hepatitis, and first in English [54] large increases in both the serum and liver aspartate and alanine transaminases in murine hepatitis. Wroblewski and LaDue were quick to recognize [55] that liver disease caused as great or great elevations of SGOT (AST) than myocardial infarction, and this was a measure of liver cell injury but not of whole liver dysfunction. It became clear that the SGPT (ALT) was generally more elevated than SGOT (AST) in acute liver injury, but many laboratories continued to assay both, and they became commonly used as monitoring or screening tests to detect early liver injury. Measurement of transaminases became the standard, and ultimately automated, way to assess hepatocellular liver injury.

Combined ALT and TBL Measurements

It was observed by Hyman J. Zimmerman,[e] after his vast experience as a consultant with hundreds of cases of liver injury caused by drugs, that hepatocellular injury

---

[e]"Hy" Zimmerman (19 July 1914–12 July 1999) was born in Rochester NY, educated there and at Stanford Medical School. He served in the army medical corps in France during World War II, where he cared for hundreds of soldiers who had fallen ill with epidemic infectious hepatitis. The experience steered him to a career in hepatology and specialization in liver injury caused by drugs or chemicals. He became one of the most beloved and respected physicians of his time, but a victim of his own pipe smoking, developing lingual carcinoma that was fatal a week short of his 85th birthday [58].

extensive enough to induce jaundice was a grave and often fatal clinical problem. He first articulated the idea in his Georgetown University Kober Lecture of 1968 [56], restated it at a Fogarty conference in 1978 [57], and reiterated it in both 1979 and 1999 editions of his book on 'Hepatotoxicity. The Adverse Effects of Drugs and Other Chemicals on the Liver'. The pithy statement that 'drug-induced hepatocellular jaundice is a serious lesion', coming from the world's most respected expert and consultant carried great weight and had much influence. These repeated opinions impressed and influenced Dr. Robert Temple of the Food and Drug Administration (FDA), who used the idea to assess hundreds of new drugs under development, and found the statement consistently true. Over Dr. Zimmerman's modest objections, Temple dubbed it 'Hy's Law' [59] at a meeting of 325 FDA medical reviewers in April 1999. The appellation caught on and stuck, and was embedded in the 2009 FDA Guidance to Industry on drug-induced liver injury [60]. That document captured the concept of 'Hy's Law' that:

> *'a finding of ALT elevation, usually substantial, seen concurrently with bilirubin > 2×ULN (Upper Limit of Normal), identifies a drug likely to cause severe DILI (Drug-Induced Liver Injury)'.*

In essence, the combined measurements became a unique 'biomarker'. However, the extent of ALT elevation that figured into 'Hy's Law' or an evaluation of DILI by itself was still given as a range.

To capture the essence of the Zimmerman observation, 'Hy's Law' if you will, and statistically evaluate the precise and temporal relationships between ALT, bilirubin and the development of DILI, a graphical statistical-medical software program, eDISH (evaluation of drug-induced serious hepatotoxicity) was developed through research under the FDA Regulatory Science Review enhancement program, by the author and Dr. Ted Guo, an experienced statistical reviewer. Starting with standardized data for the serial measurements of the serum ALT and TBL done during large clinical trials, the program displays the highest observed value for ALT on the abscissa and the highest observed TBL value on the ordinate to produce a single point for each subject studied, plotted as log10 values of the multiples above the upper limit of the normal range (ULN). Each individual point (i.e., subject) is linked to a second graphic display of all the data for that subject over the entire time of observation, allowing analysis of the temporal changes in values, and providing a detailed medical narrative to make a differential diagnosis of the likely cause.

Below is a simple graph of the basic idea: peak values (the greatest value observed at any time in the given subject, expressed as the logarithm to base 10 of multiples of the laboratory upper limit of the normal range, log10×ULN) for ALT on the abscissa and TBL on the ordinate. The use of the logarithmic scale is to keep the much greater relative elevations of ALT on the same page as those of TBL, while preserving evidence of their changes. Temple also stated that most Hy's Law cases arose out of a preponderance of ALT rises in the drug group (Temple's corollary).

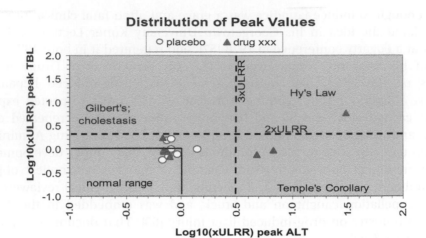

Applying this to large studies in which thousands of subjects were observed over periods of two years or more, with many observations, allows one to see at a glance the subjects with findings of highest interest, in the right upper quadrant. Subjects with points in the right upper quadrant (ALT > 3×ULN and TBL > 2×ULN) were possible Hy's Law cases, if the bilirubin rise followed ALT rise, was not mainly cholestatic, and no alternative cause was found.

Below is an eDISH plot of the time course of all liver test values (ALT, AST, ALP, TBL) for a selected subject (chosen by pointing at a symbol on the x-y plot of the log-log values). This shows the way that by inspection, much medical information may be gathered at a glance; whether the bilirubin rise followed or preceded the ALT rise, whether the ALT elevation was much greater than ALP, and whether AST was greater or less than ALT. This information then needs to be combined with a review of the narrative (available by clicking on a link on

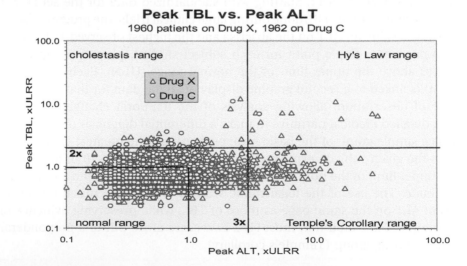

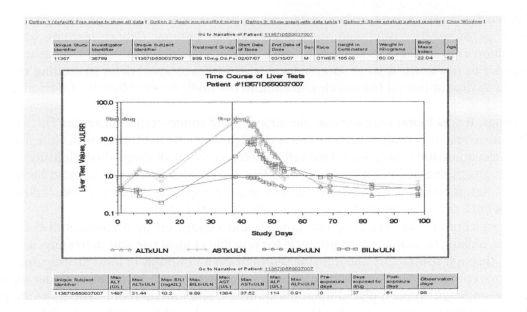

| Option 1 (default): Free scales to show all data | Option 2: Apply pre-specified scales | Option 3: Show graph with data table | Option 4: Show original patient records | Close Window |

Go to Narrative of Patient: 11357ID550037007

Unique Study Identifier	Investigator Identifier	Unique Subject Identifier	Treatment Group	Start Date of Dose	End Date of Dose	Sex	Race	Height in Centimeters	Weight in Kilograms	Body Mass Index	Age
11357	36789	11357ID550037007	B39.10mg.Od.Po	02/07/07	03/15/07	M	OTHER	165.00	60.00	22.04	52

Time Course of Liver Tests
Patient #11357ID550037007

ALTxULN   ASTxULN   ALPxULN   BILIxULN

Go to Narrative of Patient: 11357ID550037007

Unique Subject Identifier	Max ALT (U/L)	Max ALTxULN	Max BILI (mg/dL)	Max BILIxULN	Max AST (U/L)	Max ASTxULN	Max ALP (U/L)	Max ALPxULN	Pre-exposure days	Days exposed to drug	Post-exposure days	Observation days
11357ID550037007	1497	31.44	10.2	9.89	1384	37.52	114	0.91	0	37	61	98

the time course graph) to permit a physician knowledgeable about the process and art of differential diagnosis to estimate the most likely cause of the abnormalities shown.

The eDISH analysis uses the power of the computer to gather very large amounts of information as data points and to quickly display results for hundreds or thousands of individuals for selection of subjects of special interest. A second step is then to show all the information available for the selected individual, and then call up a narrative description of the case to use medical differential diagnostic reasoning to reach conclusions as to the most likely cause. The eDISH program has now been used to aid medical reviewers to assess very large clinical trials for cases of serious liver toxicity that were caused by drugs, for safety evaluation of new drugs under consideration for approval. As the serious cases are generally quite rare, not very many need detailed diagnostic assessment, yet the program pulls the needles from the haystacks. The eDISH program has been used to evaluate studies of over 14,000 and 18,000 subjects for single drug studies; it is now being considered for licensing for use outside the FDA. It has also been found useful by pharmaceutical companies seeking to obtain approval of new products by allowing their own analyses before data submission for FDA evaluation [61], and is proposed as a research tool for evaluating large databases of information concerning liver injury. Further uses of the eDISH program are under development.

Conclusions and Recommendations

It has become clear that elevations of ALT or other enzymes are not measures of the severity of hepatocellular injury, and are not sufficiently specific for diagnosis, especially for relatively rare events of low incidence or prevalence. We now propose that the gradings of severity published since 1982 by the National Cancer Institute as the Common Terminology Criteria for Adverse Events be considered instead for measures of urgency to repeat the tests at once, in local laboratories to avoid delay in sending specimens to distant central laboratories, to confirm the findings, establish the direction and rapidity of change, and to initiate additional studies to clarify the probable cause of the findings. It was found long ago that elevations in the concentration of serum TBL, or of the direct-reacting, conjugated bilirubin, were highly specific to liver problems (the much rarer elevation due to accelerated red cell hemolysis is easily distinguished clinically), but rather insensitive and often occurring only late in a disease process. It has also become clear that the search for new biomarkers must accept the combined biomarker of [ALT&TBL] rise as a standard to surpass, rather than ALT alone.

Most clinical trials are designed, funded, and conducted by pharmaceutical companies seeking to evaluate new products for possible clinical use and marketing, sometimes through contractors and utilizing scores or even hundreds of local investigators in multiple countries. The responsibility to assure the safety [62] of the products under study has recently (2010) been placed upon the sponsors, and initiation of follow-up study to determine the severity and probable cause of abnormal findings, such as possible drug-induced liver disease or dysfunction, is no longer left to the discretion of investigators, as was emphasized in a 2011 editorial [63] by members of the Center for Drug Evaluation and Research. The primary measure used to detect acute liver injury has been serum ALT, and very recent efforts have been published to establish better criteria for what constitutes levels [64] that should incite immediate repeat, follow-up, and further investigation. It is not entirely clear just how these 'classic' biomarkers have come to be so widely accepted, but it is also clear now that their use and interpretation can be misunderstood. Standardization of both methods for measurement and what constitutes truly normal ranges would be helpful.

For the present and future, it should be realized that the evolution of biomarkers for liver injury and dysfunction has taught us several lessons:

1) Elevations in serum enzyme activities do not measure function of the whole liver, but are markers of hepatocellular injury (ALT) or cholestasis (ALP).
2) Serum total bilirubin concentration is a marker of whole liver dysfunction (if not caused by accelerated heme breakdown), and is the only liver function test of the set.
3) The combined [ALT&TBL] biomarker is far more specific than ALT alone, and should be the standard against which new biomarkers for liver diseases should be compared.
4) Severity of liver disease is determined by whole organ functional loss, not by the degree of elevation of serum enzyme tests such as ALT or ALP, so the NIH/NCI gradings for severity should be replaced by the term urgency to repeat and confirm as soon as possible any reported elevations in test values.
5) Abnormalities in test values do not predict what will happen, only what has happened so far, and prompt repeat testing to confirm and find out direction and

pace of time change should be done, with supplemental investigation to diagnose the most likely cause.

6) Revision of guidances, teaching, and practice habits will need to reflect these points.

References

[1] Hijmans van den Bergh AA, Snapper I. Die Farbstoffe des Blutserums. (The colored material of serum). Deutsch Arch Klin Med 1913;110:540.

[2] Cappell MS. The effect of Naziism on medical progress in gastroenterology: The inefficiency of evil. Dig Dis Sci 2006 June; 51(6):1137–58.

[3] Ehrlich P. Sulfodiazobenzol, ein Reagenz auf Bilirubin. (Sulfodiazobenzene, a reagent for bilirubin) Zentralblatt fur klinische Medizin 1883 Nov 10; 4(45):721–3.

[4] Malloy HT, Evelyn KA. The determination of bilirubin with the photoelectric colorimeter. J Biol Chem 1937;119:437.

[5] Cremer RJ, Perryman PW, Richards DH, Holbrook B. Photosensitivity of serum bilirubin (abstract). Biochem J 1957 Aug; 66(4):60P.

[6] Schmid R. Direct-reacting bilirubin, bilirubin glucuronie, in serum, bile, and urine. Science 1956 Jul 13; 124(3211):76–7.

[7] Billing BH, Lathe GH. The excretion of bilirubin as a diglucuronide, giving the direct van den Bergh reaction (abstract, 22 March). Biochem J 1956 May;63(1):p. 6.

[8] Talafant E. Properties and composition of the bile pigment giving a direct diazo reaction. Nature 1956 Aug 11;178:312.

[9] Arias IM, London IM. Bilirubin glucuronide formation *in vitro*; demonstration of a defect in Gilbert's disease. Science 1957 Sep 20;126(3273):563–4.

[10] Gilbert A, Lereboullet P. La cholemie simple familiale. (Simple familial hyperbilirubin-emia) Semaine Med 1901;21:241.

[11] Ostrow JD, Schmid R. The protein-binding of C14-bilirubin in human and murine serum. J Clin Invest 1963 Aug;42:1286–99.

[12] Tenhunen R, Marver HS, Schmid R. The enzymatic conversion of heme to bilirubin by microsomal heme oxygenase. Proc Natl Acad Sci U S A 1968 Oct;61(2):748–85.

[13] Singleton JW, Laster L. Biliverdin reductase of guinea pig liver. J Biol Chem 1965 Dec;240(12): 4780–9.

[14] Hutchinson DW, Johnson B, Knell AJ. The reaction between bilirubin and aromatic diazo compounds. Biochem J 1972;127:907–8.

[15] Kuenzle CC, Sommenhalder M, Ruttner JR, Maier C. Separation and quantitative estimation of four bilirubin fractions from serum and of three bilirubin fractions from bile. J Lab Clin Med 1966 Feb; 67(2):282–93.

[16] Kuenzle CC, Maier C, Ruttner JR. The nature of four bilirubin fractions from serum and of three bilirubin fractions from bile. J Lab Clin Med 1966 Feb;67(2):293–306.

[17] Weiss JS, Gautam A, Lauff JJ, Sundberg MW, Jatlow P, Boyer JL, et al. The clinical importance of a protein-bound fraction of serum bilirubin in patients with hyperbilirubinemia. N Engl J Med 1983 Jul 21;308(3):147–50.

[18] Levi AJ, Gatmaitin Z, Arias IM. Two hepatic cytoplasmic protein fractions Y and Z, and their possible role in the hepatic uptake of bilirubin, sulfobromophthalein, and other anions. J Clin Invest 1969 Nov;48(11):2156–67.

[19] Ostrow JD, Mukejee P, Tiribelli C. Structure and function of unconjugated bilirubin: relevance for physiological and pathophysiological function. J Lipid Res 1994;35(10):1715–37.

[20] Fuhua P, Xuhui D, Zhiyang Z, Ying J, Yu Y, Feng T, et al. Antioxidant status of bilirubin and uric acid in patients with myasthenia gravis. Neuroimmuno-modulation 2012;19(1):43–9.

[21] Roberts WM. Variations in the phosphatase activity of the blood in disease. Br J Exper Pathol 1930; 11:90–5.

[22] Roberts WM. Blood phosphatase and the van den Bergh reaction in the differentiation of the several types of jaundice. Br Med J 1933 Apr 29;1(3773):734–8.

[23] Bodansky A. Phosphatase studies: I. Determination of inorganic phosphate. Beer's Law and interfering substances in the Kuttner-Lichtenstein method. J Biol Cem 1932 Dec;99:197–206.

[24] King EJ, Armstrong AR. A convenient method for determining serum and bile phosphatase activity. Can Med Assoc J 1934 Oct;31(4):376–81.

[25] Keay H, Trew JA. Auromated determination of serum alkaline phosphatase using a modified Bodansky technic. Clin Chem 1964 Jan;10:75–82.

[26] Report of the Commission on Enzymes of the International Union of Biochemistry. Oxford: Pergamon Press; 1961.

[27] Sebesta DG, Bradshaw FJ, Prockop DJ. Source of the elevated serum alkaline phosphatase activity in biliary obstruction; studies using isolated liver perfusion. Gastroenterology 1964 Aug;47:166–70.

[28] Senior JR, London WT, Sutnick AI. The Australia antigen and role of the late Philadelphia General Hospital in reducing post-transfusion hepatitis and sequelae. Hepatology 2011 Sep;54(3):753–6.

[29] Kaplan MM, Righetti A. Induction of rat liver alkaline phosphatase: the mechanism of the serum elevation in bile duct obstruction. J Clin Invest 1970 Mar;49(3):508–16.

[30] Polin SG, Spellberg MA, Teitelman L, Okumura M. The origin of elevation of serum alkaline phosphatase in hepatic disease. An experimental study. Gastroenterology 1962 Apr;42:431–8.

[31] Boernig H, Horn A, Mueller W. (The mechanism of change of activity of alkaline phosphatase in liver and intestine of the rat following ligation of the common bile duct.). Acta Biol Med Ger 1969; 22(3):537–49.

[32] Moss DW, Baron DN, Walker PG, Wikinson JH. Standardization of clinical enzyme assays. J Clin Pathol 1971 Nov;24(8):740–3.

[33] Hirst AD, Howorth PJN. Standardization of clinical enzyme assays. Letter to the editor. J Clin Pathol 1972 Aug;25(4):308–9.

[34] Van Wersch. On the origin of alkaline serum phosphatase after ligation of the common bile duct, with special reference to the enzyme's intrahepatic localization. Acta Anat (Basel) 1963;53:227–33.

[35] Jung W, Gebhardt R, Mecke D. Alterations in activity and ultrastructural localization of several phosphatases on the surface of adult rat hepatocytes in primary monolayer culture. Eur J Cell Biol 1982 Jun;27(2):230–41.

[36] DeBroe ME, Roels F, Nouwen EJ, Claeys L, Wieme RJ. Liver plasma membrane: the source of high molecular weight alkaline phosphatase in human serum. Hepatology 1985 Jan-Feb;5(1):118–28.

[37] Bertone V, Tarantola E, Ferrigno A, Gringneri E, Barni S, Vairetti M, et al. Altered alkaline phosphatase activity in obese Zucker rats liver with respect to lean Zucker and Wistar rats discussed in terms of all putative roles ascribed to the enzyme. Eur J Histochem 2011 Feb 8;55(1).

[38] Benichou C. Criteria of drug-induced liver disorders. Report of an international consensus meeting. J Hepatol 1990 Sep;11(2):272–6.

[39] Hanger FM. Serological differentiation of obstructive from hepatogenous jaundice by flocculation of cephalin-cholesterol emulsions. J Clin Invest 1939 May;18(3):261–9.

[40] Pohle FJ, Stewart JK. The cephalin-cholesaterol flocculation test as an aid in the diagnosis of hepatic disorders. J Clin Invest 1941 Mar;20(2):241–7.

[41] Moore DB, Pierson PS, Hanger FM, Moore DH. Mechamism of the positive cephalin-cholesterol flocculation reaction in hepatitis. J Clin Invest 1945 May;24(3):292–5.

[42] Maclagen NF. Thymol turbidity test: a new indicator of liver dysfunction. Nature 1944 Nov 25; 154(3917):670–1.

[43] Dodd DC. Use of the thymol turbidity test as an aid in diagnosis of dysfunctions of the liver. Calif Med 1947 Mar;66(3):125–7.

[44] Carter AB, Maclagen NF. Some observations on liver function tests in diseases not primarily hepatic. Br Med J 1946 Jul 20;2(4463):80–2.

[45] Rosalski SB, McIntyre N. Biochemical investigations in the management of liver disease. In: Bircher Johannes, Benhamou Jean-Pierre, McIntyre Neil, Rizzetto Mario, Rodes Juan, editors. Oxford Textbook of Clinical Hepatology (Chapter 5.1). Oxford University Press; 1999.

[46] Poynard T, Imbert-Bismut F. Laboratory testing for liver disease. In: Thomas Boyer D, Theresa Wright L, Michael Manns P, editors. Zakim and Boyer's Hepatology: A Textbook of Liver Disease (Chapter 14). 5th ed. Philadelphia PA: Elsevier Inc; 2006.

[47] Ozer JS, Chetty R, Kenna G, Koppiker N, Karamjeet P, Li D, et al. Recommendations to qualify biomarker candidates of drug-induced liver injury. Biomark Med 2010 Jun;$(3):475–83.

[48] Karmen A. A note on the spectrophotometic assay of glutamic-oxalacetic transaminase in human blood serum. J Clin Invest 1955 Jan;34:131–3.

[49] Karmen A, Wroblewski F, LaDue JS. Transaminase activity in human blood. J Clin Invest 1955 Jan; 34:126–31.

[50] Wroblewski F, LaDue JS. Myocardial infarction as a post-operative complication of major surgery. J Am Med Assoc 1952 Nov 22;150(12):1212–6.

[51] LaDue JS, Wroblewski F, Karmen A. Serum glutamic oxalacetic transaminase activity in human acute transmural myocardial infarction. Science 1954 Sep 24;120(3117):497–9.

[52] Wroblewski F, LaDue JS. Serum glutamic oxalacetic transaminase activity as an index of liver cell injury: a preliminary report. Ann Intern Med 1955 Aug;43(2):345–60.

[53] Reitman S, Frankel S. A colorimetric method for the determination of serum glutamic oxalacetic and glutamic pyruvic transaminases. Am J Clin Pathol 1957 Jul;28(1):56–63.

[54] De Ritis F, Coltori M, Giusti G. Serum and liver transaminase activities in experimental viral hepatitis in mice. Science 1956 Jul 6;124(3210):32.

[55] Wroblewski F, LaDue JS. Serum glutamic oxalacetic transaminase activity as an index of liver cell injury: a preliminary report. Ann Intern Med 1955 Aug;43(2):345–60.

[56] Zimmerman HJ. The spectrum of hepatotoxicity. Perspect Biol Med 1968;12(1):135–61.

[57] Davidson CS, Leevy CM, Chamberlayne EC, editors. Guidelines for the detection of hepatotoxicity due to drugs and chemicals. US Department of Health, Education, and Welfare, Public Health Service. National Institutes of Health. NIH Publication; 1979. p. 79–313.

[58] Seeff LB, Hyman J, Zimmerman MD. J Am Med Assoc 2000 Feb 9;283(6):812.

[59] Reuben A. Hy's Law. Hepatology 2004 Feb;39(2):574–8.

[60] Center for Drug Evaluation and Research/Center for Biologics Evaluation and Research. Drug-induced liver injury; premarketing clinical evaluation (guidance document). Food and Drug Administration, US Department of Health and Human Services July 2009.

[61] Watkins PB, Desai M, Berkowitz SD, Peters G, Horsmans Y, Larrey D, et al. Evaluation of drug-induced serious hepatotoxicity (eDISH): application of this data organization approach to

phase III clinical trial of rivaroxban after total hip or knee replacement surgery. Drug Safety 2011 Mar 1;34(3):243–52.

[62] FDA. Investigational new drug safety reporting requirements for human drug and biological products and safety reporting requirements for bioavailability and bioequivalence studies in humans: final rule. Fed Regist 2010;75(188):59935–63.

[63] Sherman RB, Woodcock J, Norden J, Grandinetti C, Temple RJ. New FDA regulation to improve safety reporting in clinical trials. N Engl J Med 2011 Jul 7;365(1):3–5.

[64] Ruhl CE, Everhart JE. Upper limits of normal for alanine aminotransferase activity in the United States population. Hepatology 2012 Feb;55(2):447–54.

14

Qualification of Urinary Biomarkers for Kidney Toxicity

Joseph V. Bonventre[1], Vishal S. Vaidya[1,2]

[1]RENAL DIVISION, DEPARTMENT OF MEDICINE, BRIGHAM AND WOMEN'S HOSPITAL, BOSTON, MASSACHUSETTS, USA, [2]HARVARD SCHOOL OF PUBLIC HEALTH, BOSTON, MASSACHUSETTS, USA

Regulatory Framework: Advancing the Science of Biomarkers

In 2004, the US Food and Drug Administration (FDA) launched its Critical Path Initiative. Recognizing the increasingly complicated and difficult path to medical product development, the FDA concluded that it was very important to develop new tools to evaluate and predict the safety, efficacy and manufacturability of medical products. The FDA called for a national effort to identify specific activities all along the critical path of medical product development and use, which, if undertaken, would help transform the critical path sciences.

The Critical Path Initiative reinforced the need for additional biomarkers to predict drug toxicity in pre-clinical studies which can act as surrogate endpoints, and/or aid in making efficacious and cost-saving decisions or terminating drug development more quickly [1]. It was predicted that quantifiable and sensitive biomarkers would influence every phase of the drug development process, from discovery and pre-clinical evaluation through each phase of clinical trials and post-marketing studies.

With the advent of 'omics' technology, discovering/identifying potentially useful biomarkers for a particular disease state has become more pervasive over the last two decades, but establishing the utility of these putative tools remains very challenging. Furthermore, the utility of a particular biomarker may be very 'context-specific'. The importance of the contextual aspect of evaluation of the utility of the marker was reflected by the process of evaluation as well as the terminology. While the 'validation' of a biomarker assay measurement test is an important process, the regulatory agencies focus on biomarker validity in a particular context or contexts, and generally use the term 'qualification' as relating to the context for which the biomarker is proven to be valid [2]. The extensive nature of biomarker evaluation demands an organized, systematic and structured outcome-oriented approach, and the kind of science that moves away from a traditional one-lab-one-project-one-publication type of thinking. This is exactly what the

The Path from Biomarker Discovery to Regulatory Qualification. http://dx.doi.org/10.1016/B978-0-12-391496-5.00014-4

FDA qualification process did. It set a regulatory framework to guide investigators in most expeditiously moving the early biomarker observations to the next phase that would have the highest impact in science and medicine.

Kidney Injury Molecule-1: Characteristics

We became involved in the qualification process through an invitation to work with the Predictive Safety Testing Consortium (PSTC), organized by the non-profit Critical Path Institute (C-Path). The consortium was very interested in Kidney Injury Molecule-1 (KIM-1 in rodents and humans) as one of the urinary biomarkers that they initially considered. We had already been collaborating scientifically with members of the FDA toxicology laboratory in examining the performance of KIM-1 in models of injury that they were working on. We first reported KIM-1 in 1998 [3] as a putative epithelial cell adhesion molecule containing a novel immunoglobulin domain, which is markedly up-regulated in renal cells after injury. In this and subsequent studies it was demonstrated that this protein was increased in expression in the proximal tubule of the kidney after multiple forms of injury, more so than any other protein. KIM-1 is a type I cell membrane glycoprotein, which contains extracellular immunoglobulin and N- and O-glycosylation mucin-like domains, as well as a transmembrane and short intracellular domains. KIM-1 is a phosphatidylserine receptor that recognizes apoptotic cells, directing them to lysosomes [4]. It also is a receptor for oxidized lipoproteins. KIM-1 is unique in being the first molecule, not also present on myeloid cells, that transforms kidney proximal epithelial cells into semi-professional phagocytes [4,5].

The KIM-1 protein is expressed on the apical membrane of proximal tubule cells and its ectodomain is cleaved and released into the lumen of the tubule [6]. Once our laboratory recognized this ectodomain release [6], we determined that it was mediated by metalloproteases and then determined that it was present in the urine of patients with various forms of kidney injury [7]. We subsequently confirmed that the ectodomain was very stable in urine, making it useful as a marker of kidney injury. We performed a large number of animal studies, which demonstrated a very good correlation between kidney injury due to multiple causes and urinary levels of KIM-1. Many of these were performed in collaboration with other laboratories. Some of the causes of injury in these studies included: ischemia reperfusion, cisplatin, S-(1,1,2,2-tetrafluoroethyl)-l-cysteine (TFEC), cadmium [8,9], folic acid [10], gentamicin, mercury, chromium [11], vancomycin, ochratoxin A, cyclosporine [12], iodinated contrast agents [13], d-serine, donor brain death induced kidney injury prior to transplantation [14], protein overload nephropathy [15] and aging-induced nephropathy.

Up to 2006, the diagnostic ability of KIM-1 as a biomarker was evaluated to significantly advance our understanding of its reproducibility, translatability and early diagnostic ability. At the same time we explored the biology of the molecule. Our approach was methodical with careful development of monoclonal antibodies that would be highly specific and sensitive. We spent a great deal of time establishing assays before rushing to publish because of our concern that bad assays would contaminate the literature – a concern that has been borne out in other biomarker studies. We developed a very reproducible assay on the Luminex platform, and tested it for a number of potentially interfering agents. We developed assays for the rat and human. We characterized KIM-1 expression and urinary excretion in a large number of toxicity studies in our lab and in collaboration with many other labs throughout the world, including those in the Center for Devices and Radiological Health at the FDA. Once the human assay was established as reliable, we began to publish findings in humans and began to measure KIM-1 levels in the urine of individuals throughout the world.

Collaborations in Consortia

We were initially asked to collaborate in another pre-clinical consortium, and were happy to do so until there were barriers established because we had not yet commercialized the assay. The members of the consortium felt that they did not want to study biomarkers that were not commercially available. We had strategically decided not to license KIM-1 and its assay to any one company, but rather to license it to a number of companies so that competition would be possible and the price would then ultimately be compatible with a high level of usage in patients – which was the main reason we were spending a great deal of effort characterizing the protein and validating reliable assays.

We were very pleased to be asked to be part of the PSTC, formed as a result of the FDA initiative regarding the regulatory framework around biomarker qualification. The PSTC did not consider the absence of a commercialized assay a problem, since, as stated in a review co-authored by Drs. Goodsaid and Frueh of the FDA and Mattes of the Critical Path Institute:

> '...there is an excellent chance that if it is a novel biomarker there will be no off-the-shelf tests available for it.' [16]

This open collaboration of individuals representing 17 pharmaceutical/biotechnology companies, regulatory bodies and academia engaged in a rigorous evaluation of both the status of biomarker science, as well as a mechanism to explore processes that would optimize content and structure presentation of that content to regulatory bodies for review. One of us (JVB) met with Dr. Goodsaid, who was representing the FDA in this initiative and who served as a strong advocate of the process. He emphasized that the consortium was interested in having KIM-1 included in the list of biomarkers that would be tested, and, since the PSTC wanted to be at the cutting edge of biomarker evaluation, did not want to exclude promising biomarkers that were in earlier stages of development or commercialization, as long as there was a reliable assay. KIM-1's performance was tested in over 13 mechanistically distinct animal models of kidney toxicity in a large number of biological specimens collected from various time points from rats receiving various doses of toxins. Most of the samples were obtained from companies represented by members of the consortium. We were asked to transfer our analytical reagents to a commercial company who would do the assays for the consortium. We agreed to do so, and also worked with that company to validate their use of the assay. While most of the assays were carried out by this company, we also continued to perform assays on samples provided by the FDA research laboratories obtained from rats treated with gentamicin, mercuric chloride or chromium [11], as well as samples from rats treated with varying times of ischemia in the laboratory of Dr. Norma Bobadilla from Mexico City [17]. We were blinded to the characteristics of all the biological samples we analyzed.

Interactions with the FDA and EMA

We found the PSTC to be a motivated group of individuals who were on a mission: to find biomarkers of kidney safety that would enable drug development. For much of the time we were the only academic representatives in the consortium. We rapidly became accustomed to the 'Pharma' way which this group had of dealing with the challenge at hand: be efficient, be collaborative, be rigorous and keep the FDA and EMA qualification process always in site. We also came to understand how the regulatory agencies perceived the process and success. The FDA and EMA developed efficient processes, and in 2003 agreed for the first time to allow the option for sponsors to have joint FDA-EMA voluntary genomic data submission (VGDS) [2]. We attended a number of meetings at the FDA headquarters, presented our findings on the use of biomarkers in a number of models of kidney disease as well as in patients with various types of kidney diseases. The discussions were always lively and very instructive for us, as they helped to focus on the very important issues that were necessary to address in order for a biomarker to be accepted into general usage. Often the meetings were teleconferenced with the EMA, and sometimes with the Japanese regulatory agency. The regulatory agencies were keen to encourage public–private partnerships and consortia. The goal was to generate data that could be pooled and result in a critical mass of information that would increase our understanding of biomarkers and how they behave in various related and unrelated conditions [2]. There was a good deal of discussion about the important differences between 'qualification' and 'validation' of a biomarker, terms that are frequently inappropriately used interchangeably. As discussed previously, validation applies to the assay: what is the assay reliability and what is the range over which it is reliable in the context of the purpose for which the assay will be used? Qualification is the result of evaluation of evidence that leads to a conclusion that a biomarker can be linked to a biological process or clinical endpoint in a fit-for-purpose context [18].

The voluntary exploratory data submission (VXDS) was initiated in June of 2007 and included seven urinary biomarkers, including KIM-1, clusterin, albumin, total protein, β2-microglobulin, cystatin C and trefoil factor 3 (TFF3). There were a number of subsequent communications among members of the PSTC and the FDA and EMA. Evidence was presented that KIM-1, clusterin, TTF3 and albumin, as tubular injury markers, and total protein, β2 microglobulin and cystatin C as markers for alteration or damage of glomeruli outperformed blood urea nitrogen (BUN) and serum creatinine (SCr) as early diagnostic indicators of drug-induced nephrotoxicity in rats. In addition to recommending that these markers in rat studies, along with TFF3, be individually qualified for regulatory decision-making, the PSTC also recommended that the biomarkers could also be useful in the clinical translational context. After much discussion and modifications of the VXDS, on June 12, 2008 the FDA and EMA jointly announced qualification of the urinary biomarkers. This was historic in that it represented for the first time a joint response of the FDA and EMA to a single submission to the two agencies. It also represented the first time that a group of drug companies worked together to collect the evidence and propose new safety tests jointly to the FDA and EMA. The FDA and EMA came to the conclusions that:

- The seven kidney biomarkers are acceptable in the context of non-clinical drug development for the detection of acute drug-induced kidney toxicity.
- The kidney biomarkers provide additional and complementary information to the currently available standards.
- The use of kidney biomarkers in clinical trials is to be considered on a case-by-case basis in order to gather further data to qualify their usefulness in monitoring drug-induced kidney toxicity in humans.

This qualification process has had a major impact on the evaluation of the safety of drugs in development. A very important, and inadequately appreciated, conclusion of the PSTC was that urinary albumin was an excellent marker of kidney tubular injury. Urinary albumin is traditionally considered a marker for glomerular disease. There is currently a good deal of controversy regarding the amount of albumin that escapes the glomerular filter under normal conditions and it has been appreciated that the proximal tubule can take up albumin from the lumen, but it nevertheless has been considered that increases in urinary albumin are most reflective of glomerular disease. The PSTC data analysis revealed that the traditional view should be challenged. Proximal tubular cell injury likely limits the tubular capacity to reabsorb albumin. Hence urinary albumin, a readily available test, may be very useful in patients if one can have access to baseline measurements and can monitor values over time. Another surprising conclusion of the consortium was that β2-microglobulin, a 'legacy' biomarker widely considered a marker of tubule injury [19], was actually found to be a biomarker for glomerular injury. Lastly, although it has been long recognized that the traditional markers such as blood urea nitrogen and serum creatinine are insensitive, delayed and non-specific biomarkers, this consortium demonstrated for the first time these shortcomings very effectively using the most comprehensive approach taken to date. For example, the sensitivity of serum creatinine (SCr) was only 0.20 for histology grades 0 to 1 (subtle damage) and increased to only 0.56 with severity grades of 0 to 3, while urinary Kim-1 was highly sensitive and specific for assessing even the most subtle forms of proximal tubular damage (histology grade 0 to 1).

A great deal of effort was put into presenting the results of the consortium in a comprehensive but readable fashion in a set of original articles and reviews, published in *Nature Biotechnology* in May 2010. Data presented in the manuscript on the performance of KIM-1 [20] demonstrated that it outperformed BUN, SCr and urinary NAG, and achieved an area under the curve for the receiver operating characteristic curve (ROC-AUC) of 0.91 to 0.99. The AUC for KIM-1 remained greater than 0.9 whether the entire histopathology spectrum was included or whether the analyzed group was restricted to low grades of histopathology. A threshold increase of 1.87-fold increase in urinary KIM-1 concentration for 95% specificity derived from one laboratory was similarly and independently defined in other laboratories using other study designs for kidney injury. This was the first report clearly documenting that BUN and SCr were useful only with more severe histopathological grades in pre-clinical studies of nephrotoxicity.

Translation to Clinical Use

A key aspect of the consortium was the careful attention to pathology as the gold standard for measuring biomarker performance. In order to use histopathology as the gold standard it was necessary that the consortium should standardize the assessment, to ensure specificity, sensitivity, objectivity and consistency. The pathologists developed a standardized lexicon and grading structure [21]. This lexicon was organized by anatomical location of the histological lesions to the cortex, medulla, papillae or renal pelvis. Within each of the localizations there was a sublocalization (e.g., glomerulus, proximal tubule (S1,2 or S3 segment), loop of Henle, thick ascending limb, distal convoluted tubule, collecting duct). The lesions were characterized as: necrosis, apoptosis, basophilia, increased mitosis, hyaline droplet formation, hypertrophy, nuclear change, cellular sloughing, pigmentation accumulation, vacuolation, tubular dilatation or cystic dilatation. Any casts present were described and any vascular, perivascular and interstitial lesions described using a standardized lexicon. This careful attention to the detail of the lesions was critical for an adequate evaluation of the biomarkers and was one of the reasons why the consortium was so successful.

This is in stark contrast to what is possible in human studies designed for biomarker qualification. Serum creatinine concentration (SCr) is the test used for the diagnosis of kidney injury in humans, and relative or absolute changes in SCr are used to score the severity of acute kidney injury. SCr is acknowledged, however, to be an inadequate gold standard for several reasons. It has poor specificity in settings where there is decrease in glomerular filtration rate without injury, such as can occur with changes in kidney blood flow or changes in dietary intake. Furthermore, drug-induced changes in the tubular secretion of creatinine may lead to changes in SCr without actual injury to the kidney being present [22]. SCr has poor sensitivity in the setting where baseline kidney function is very good and there is a large amount of renal reserve [23]. SCr may not change even if injury is present, because of compensatory increases in function by other nephrons, and also because SCr is not very sensitive to changes in kidney function at near normal levels of function. The consortium fortunately did not have to rely on SCr in the rat because of the ready availability of kidney tissue to evaluate. In fact, the PSTC found that KIM-1 was prodromal as a biomarker, increasing in the urine at a time before histopathology became apparent.

Despite the inadequacies of SCr, clinical studies continue to use changes in SCr as the 'gold standard' against which to test novel tubular injury biomarkers. This has led to studies in which the AUC-ROC are significantly lower than the levels in pre-clinical studies and, in our opinion, represents the largest hurdle to progress in the use of kidney safety markers in humans [24]. Long term outcome studies will take a number of years to conduct. Many of the participants in the PSTC are considering the pursuit of a cisplatin nephrotoxicity study in patients with head and neck tumors. Most of these patients will have normal renal function at baseline with a great deal of 'renal reserve'. This will result in injury without changes in SCr and also changes in SCr, associated with volume depletion associated with response to chemotherapy, without necessarily tubular injury. On the other hand, one would expect that there will be significantly more increases seen in urinary biomarkers of injury in the cisplatin treated group as compared to the control group (radiation treatment without cisplatin). At some point, however, in our opinion we will have to disengage from the use of SCr as a gold standard and interpret the response of biomarkers in humans as reflecting the pathology seen in rats, mice and other experimental animals. Multiple biomarkers can be used initially to reassure us that we can rely on the signals that are being generated. While histopathology in a subset of human cases may be helpful, it will never be adequate to completely resolve the gold standard problem due to the limited number of patient biopsies and limited amount of tissue from those patients biopsied. It is important to understand the specificity of the biomarkers. Specific kidney injury markers will possibly be most reliably used initially for their negative predictive value, in the context of the patient receiving nephrotoxicants. If the biomarker(s) is(are) not increased then it is unlikely that a change in SCr is related to injury. The nephrotoxicant can then be continued or its dose can be increased if deemed clinically desirable.

Conclusions

The urinary biomarker qualification process that we were involved in over a number of years was a very rewarding experience, which proved to be educational in a number of ways: we gained a better understanding of the regulatory process, and an appreciation of the effectiveness of consortia that are agile, motivated, focused, can move quickly, and are populated by individuals who work well together. One of the key success stories for the regulatory framework that functioned for qualification is that it allowed most effective and efficient international collaboration between industry, regulatory agencies and academics in a precompetitive space providing major scientific advances that otherwise would not have happened. Hopefully the continuing process will lead to improved patient safety and more efficient therapeutic development.

References

[1] Challenge and opportunity on the critical path to new medical products. In: US FDA. http://www.fda.gov/oc/initiatives/criticalpath/whitepaper.html; 2004.

[2] Goodsaid F, Papaluca M. Evolution of biomarker qualification at the health authorities. Nat Biotechnol 2010;28:441–3.

[3] Ichimura T, Bonventre JV, Bailly V, Wei H, Hession CA, Cate RL, et al. Kidney injury molecule-1 (KIM-1), a putative epithelial cell adhesion molecule containing a novel immunoglobulin domain, is up-regulated in renal cells after injury. J Biol Chem 1998;273:4135–42.

[4] Ichimura T, Asseldonk EJ, Humphreys BD, Gunaratnam L, Duffield JS, Bonventre JV. Kidney injury molecule-1 is a phosphatidylserine receptor that confers a phagocytic phenotype on epithelial cells. J Clin Invest 2008;118:1657–68.

[5] Savill J, Fadok V. Corpse clearance defines the meaning of cell death. Nature 2000;407:784–8.

[6] Bailly V, Zhang Z, Meier W, Cate R, Sanicola M, Bonventre JV. Shedding of kidney injury molecule-1, a putative adhesion protein involved in renal regeneration. J Biol Chem 2002;277:39739–48.

[7] Han WK, Bailly V, Abichandani R, Thadhani R, Bonventre JV. Kidney injury molecule-1 (KIM-1): a novel biomarker for human renal proximal tubule injury. Kidney Int 2002;62:237–44.

[8] Prozialeck WC, Vaidya VS, Liu J, Waalkes MP, Edwards JR, Lamar PC, et al. Kidney injury molecule-1 is an early biomarker of cadmium nephrotoxicity. Kidney Int 2007;72:985–93.

[9] Prozialeck WC. Toxicology and Applied Pharmacology. Foreword. Toxicol Appl Pharmacol 2009; 238:191.

[10] Ichimura T, Hung CC, Yang SA, Stevens JL, Bonventre JV. Kidney injury molecule-1: a tissue and urinary biomarker for nephrotoxicant-induced renal injury. Am J Physiol Renal Physiol 2004;286: F552–63.

[11] Zhou Y, Vaidya VS, Brown RP, Zhang J, Rosenzweig BA, Thompson KL, et al. Comparison of kidney injury molecule-1 and other nephrotoxicity biomarkers in urine and kidney following acute exposure to gentamicin, mercury, and chromium. Toxicol Sci 2008;101:159–70.

[12] Perez-Rojas J, Blanco JA, Cruz C, Trujillo J, Vaidya VS, Uribe N, et al. Mineralocorticoid receptor blockade confers renoprotection in preexisting chronic cyclosporine nephrotoxicity. Am J Physiol Renal Physiol 2007;292:F131–9.

[13] Jost G, Pietsch H, Sommer J, Sandner P, Lengsfeld P, Seidensticker P, et al. Retention of iodine and expression of biomarkers for renal damage in the kidney after application of iodinated contrast media in rats. Invest Radiol 2009. In Press.

[14] Nijboer WN, Schuurs TA, Damman J, van Goor H, Vaidya VS, van der Heide JJ, et al. Kidney injury molecule-1 is an early noninvasive indicator for donor brain death-induced injury prior to kidney transplantation. Am J Transplant 2009;9:1752–9.

[15] van Timmeren MM, Bakker SJ, Vaidya VS, Bailly V, Schuurs TA, Damman J, et al. Tubular kidney injury molecule-1 in protein-overload nephropathy. Am J Physiol Renal Physiol 2006;291:F456–64.

[16] Goodsaid FM, Frueh FW, Mattes W. Strategic paths for biomarker qualification. Toxicology 2008; 245:219–23.

[17] Vaidya VS, Ramirez V, Ichimura T, Bobadilla NA, Bonventre JV. Urinary kidney injury molecule-1: a sensitive quantitative biomarker for early detection of kidney tubular injury. Am J Physiol Renal Physiol 2006;290:F517–29.

[18] Wagner JA. Strategic approach to fit-for-purpose biomarkers in drug development. Annu Rev Pharmacol Toxicol 2008;48:631–51.

[19] Trof RJ, Di Maggio F, Leemreis J, Groeneveld AB. Biomarkers of acute renal injury and renal failure. Shock 2006;26:245–53.

[20] Vaidya VS, Ozer JS, Dieterle F, Collings FB, Ramirez V, Troth S, et al. Kidney injury molecule-1 outperforms traditional biomarkers of kidney injury in pre-clinical biomarker qualification studies. Nat Biotechnol 2010;28:478–85.

[21] Sistare FD, Dieterle F, Troth S, Holder DJ, Gerhold D, Andrews-Cleavenger D, et al. Towards consensus practices to qualify safety biomarkers for use in early drug development. Nat Biotechnol 2010;28:446–54.

[22] Blantz RC. Pathophysiology of pre-renal azotemia. Kidney Int 1998;53:512–23.

[23] Bosch JP, Saccaggi A, Lauer A, Ronco C, Belledonne M, Glabman S. Renal functional reserve in humans. Effect of protein intake on glomerular filtration rate. Am J Med 1983;75:943–50.

[24] Waikar SS, Betensky RA, Emerson SC, Bonventre JV. Imperfect gold standards for kidney injury biomarker evaluation. J Am Soc Nephrol 2012;23:13–21.

Consortia

15

Renal Biomarker Qualification: An ILSI Health and Environmental Sciences Institute Perspective

Syril Pettit[1], Ernie Harpur[2]

[1]HEALTH AND ENVIRONMENTAL SCIENCES INSTITUTE (HESI), WASHINGTON DC, USA,
[2]INSTITUTE OF CELLULAR MEDICINE, NEWCASTLE UNIVERSITY, NEWCASTLE, UK

Safety Biomarker Research – the Origin of this Activity in HESI

As a result of an increasing recognition of a dearth of translational safety biomarkers, the concept for an International Life Sciences Institute (ILSI) Health and Environmental Sciences Institute (HESI) collaborative biomarker research program was developed in 2002. HESI is a non-profit, international, scientific organization based in Washington, DC, which brings academic, government, and industry scientists together through scientific research to improve drug and chemical safety evaluation. This project was driven by a shared awareness across the pharmaceutical industry, research, and regulatory communities of the limited data on the sensitivity, specificity, and translational relevance of existing biomarkers. Together these factors contributed to a potentially significant barrier to the clinical development of candidate medicines that exhibited organ toxicity in pre-clinical studies. At the same time, there was a growing conviction that the evolving 'omic' technologies had the potential to aid the discovery of new biomarkers. This was reinforced by the HESI collaborative scientific program coordinated through the Committee on the Application of Genomics to Mechanism-Based Risk Assessment (1999–2003; see vignette on this topic) where the value of transcriptomic studies in the identification of putative biomarkers of toxicity was demonstrated [1,2]. Additionally, in 2000 the Food and Drug Administration (FDA) Non-Clinical Studies Subcommittee (Advisory Committee for Pharmaceutical Sciences) undertook to examine how scientific collaboration among FDA, industry, academia and the public could be fostered in order to provide advice on improved scientific approaches to regulatory non-clinical drug development. One of two initial areas of focus identified was biomarkers of toxicity; subsequent literature reviews by FDA Expert Working Groups, such as that on Biomarkers of Drug-Induced Cardiac Toxicity [3], highlighted the problem of biomarker improvement and advocated experimental steps through which it could be addressed. These

The Path from Biomarker Discovery to Regulatory Qualification. http://dx.doi.org/10.1016/B978-0-12-391496-5.00015-6

Table 15.1   Objectives of the Proposed Activity on Biomarkers

---

1. Engage in a broad-based, multinational collaborative research program to advance the development and application of biomarkers of target organ toxicity.
2. Identify accessible biomarkers with the potential to bridge from the pre-clinical to the clinical stages of drug development.
3. Evaluate the potential utility of newly identified markers of tissue injury for pre-clinical safety studies.
4. Build consensus regarding how to apply newly identified biomarkers of toxicity in risk assessment.
5. Provide an ongoing scientific forum to facilitate discussion of the evolving state of the science related to biomarkers and proteomic technologies.

Expert Working Groups were comprised of representatives from academia, the pharmaceutical industry, the FDA and the US National Institute of Environmental Health Sciences (NIEHS), a tripartite structure that parallels that of HESI.

HESI accordingly proposed to establish a new program of activities with several objectives (Table 15.1). To this end a Biomarker Subcommittee on the Development and Application on Biomarkers of Toxicity was formed and met for the first time in November, 2002. The objectives identified at this initial meeting are shown in Table 15.2.

The output of this meeting placed primacy on the development and validation of assays for selected non-clinical biomarkers. Participants at this meeting would be invited to nominate candidate biomarkers for assay development. In line with the *modus operandi* of HESI, it was envisaged that the process would culminate in a release of information to the broader scientific community via peer-reviewed publications and/or a scientific workshop. At the time there was no process for review of biomarker data by either FDA or the European Medicines Authority (EMA) which would result in a formal opinion as to the potential utility of the biomarkers in the context of drug development (subsequently referred to as 'Qualification for Use'). FDA and other regulatory agency scientists were, however, actively involved in the HESI committee as members from its inception. The government participants in the HESI subcommittee advocated the submission of the validation data to the Interagency Coordinating Committee on the

Table 15.2   Objectives Identified at the Inaugural Meeting of the Biomarker Subcommittee on the Development and Application on Biomarkers of Toxicity

---

1. Review the utility of current biomarkers of cell and tissue damage and develop a consensus about the feasibility and value of developing improved biomarkers as an acceptable paradigm for bridging pre-clinical and clinical studies.
2. Identify specific areas of new biology and technology that could be applied to develop an improved set of appropriate biomarkers for practical application.
3. Establish which biomarkers should be examined (prioritized) and which technologies should be used.
4. Establish the optimal experimental design(s) to evaluate/validate.
5. Develop a consensus regarding whether HESI is an appropriate organization to undertake the identification and development of improved accessible biomarkers.
6. Identify a specific plan for implementing a collaborative approach to the development of such biomarkers. Survey stake holders to determine how the HESI effort might be leveraged.

Validation of Alternative Methods (ICCVAM)[1] as a means of generating a formal regulatory response to the data. The advice to prepare and submit validation data to ICCVAM was influential in the direction and design of the subsequent experimental program. As a consequence, emphasis was placed on all aspects of biomarker quantification, including detailed validation of the assays to be applied in several laboratories of the committee members (to assess inter-laboratory as well as inter-assay variability). Inevitably this required the use of extensive resources and resulted in slower progress than might otherwise have been the case. With hindsight, a lighter assay validation phase (ensuring that the assays were fit for research use in individual laboratories) would have been sufficient to progress more rapidly in the generation of biomarker data from toxicity studies and allow evaluation of diagnostic utility of the biomarkers. If individual biomarkers had shown diagnostic utility, then a second phase of rigorous assay validation could have been conducted to support further study and application of these biomarkers.

Creation of Biomarker Working Groups

At a meeting of the Biomarker Committee in July 2003, seven biomarker research proposals were critically reviewed. Taking account of numerous factors such as need, feasibility and ultimate impact including potential to bridge from pre-clinical to clinical phases of drug development, three proposals were selected for action, covering examination of biomarkers of cardiac, testicular and kidney injury. The cardiac group elected to focus on the assessment of cardiac troponin as a biomarker with known relevance in the clinic (for assessment of myocardial infarction) but limited data in the pre-clinical context. The testicular marker group sought to develop and validate rodent assays for Inhibin B – a marker thought to be associated with male fertility. Ultimately it was the kidney group, subsequently referred to here as the Biomarkers of Nephrotoxicity Committee (BNC), which made a biomarker qualification submission to FDA and EMA so the rest of this article focuses on the activities of that group.

Biomarkers of Nephrotoxicity Committee (BNC)

Development of an experimental program by the BNC was guided by the initial objectives agreed by the Biomarker Subcommittee overall (Table 15.2) and the BNC specifically. The program adopted the following general principles and approaches in its study design:

1) Compounds were selected based upon the expectation that they would cause damage to specific portions of the nephron. As far as possible, the model

---

[1]ICCVAM is comprised of representatives from fifteen government agencies. Administrative and scientific support for ICCVAM comes from the National Toxicology Program Interagency Center for Evaluation of Alternative Toxicological Methods (NICEATM) which is located in National Institute of Environmental Health Sciences (NIEHS) in Research Triangle Park, North Carolina.

compounds would represent different chemical classes, have different biological/pharmacological properties and cause renal injury by different mechanisms (where this information was available). The objective of these selection criteria was to permit the detection of renal injury irrespective of the precise nature of the chemical or the pathogenesis of the injury.

2) Male Han Wistar (HW) and Sprague Dawley (SD) rats were selected as the initial test species. Rats are the species most extensively studied in investigations of nephrotoxicity and the standard rodent species used in pre-clinical safety assessment. Both the HW and SD strains of rat are commonly used in pharmaceutical development. Dogs were not included in this first phase of the work as this was considered impractical for a variety of reasons, not least being the lack of suitable biomarker assays. As such, it was also recognized that consideration of the bridging aspects of this work would have to rely on published data in the first instance.

3) Candidate biomarkers with promise based on literature and previous HESI programs were selected as priority targets. The selection was made with consideration of the practicality of developing robust analytical methodologies. Based on precedent, urine was selected as a relevant and accessible fluid.

4) Pilot studies were conducted to define doses ranging from no observable effect dose to markedly toxic (i.e., using dose–response information to obviate the need for 'negative' controls other than vehicle).

5) Procedures were defined for sample collection by each participating laboratory to ensure optimal preservation of biomarkers and other analytes based upon best in-house practices.

6) Biomarker assays were developed where none existed previously. Newly developed assays were to be comprehensively validated with attention to accuracy, sensitivity, robustness and reproducibility within and among laboratories over time.

7) Novel biomarker data would be compared with the results of established tests or traditional biomarkers used to monitor renal injury.

8) Single definitive studies for each selected nephrotoxin and rat strain would be designed and conducted. However, urine samples from these studies were to be distributed across six labs as part of a robust assay validation process.

9) Histopathological characterization of the renal injury would be used as the definitive comparator. To enable this, a pathology working group was established to agree upon nomenclature and to peer review study results.

10) All studies were to be conducted according to Good Laboratory Practices Guidelines with the following exceptions:

   i. There would be no independent audit although each participating laboratory would be responsible for conducting thorough quality control of their data.

   ii. No formulation analysis or exposure assessment would be done since development of validated assays would require disproportionate resource and time.

Variations which occurred during the execution of the studies reflected variance in standard practice in different laboratories, and was considered to provide 'real world' context. None of these variations was judged to have compromised the objectives of the program of work or the technical rigor of the study. Cross-study comparisons were facilitated by relating all biomarker responses to histopathological changes (the diagnoses of which were harmonized across studies) and expressing all biomarker levels as fold-change from time-matched control animals of the same strain. These measures provided a high level of confidence in the multi-site data set.

The nephronal segments of particular interest to the BNC were the proximal tubule (PT), the most common target for nephrotoxic drugs, and the collecting duct (CD), a segment for which no biomarkers existed. Based on this, the initial selection of biomarker candidates to be evaluated included α- and μ-glutathione s-transferases (GST) (biomarkers of PT and distal tubular injury, respectively), Kidney Injury Molecule-1 (KIM-1) (PT), Renal Papillary Antigen-1 (RPA-1) (CD) and clusterin (no specific location in the nephron). Anticipating ICCVAM review of the protocols and data, the BNC felt it was critical to have a robust assay that could be applied in <u>all</u> of the participating laboratories to assess inter-assay reproducibility. Commercial assay kits were available from Biotrin (subsequently Argutus Medical) for the GSTs and an assay kit for RPA-1 was under development. The situation regarding KIM-1 was unclear, both from a legal (patent) perspective and the availability of a suitable antibody to allow the development of a rat assay, and could not be resolved in a reasonable timeframe. As a result, the BNC was forced to exclude KIM-1 as one of the candidate biomarkers. A potential barrier also arose to the development and use of a clusterin assay with the discovery of a broad-based patent owned by Novartis. Following legal advice and dialogue with Novartis a release document was negotiated which permitted the inclusion of clusterin in the panel of biomarkers to be evaluated. Suitable antibodies were sourced which enabled the development of a clusterin assay by Biotrin.

In parallel with the above efforts to define the group's freedom to operate and to develop suitable assays, the BNC established a process for selection of candidate nephrotoxicants for use in *in vivo* studies. While, a large number of nephrotoxic compounds were initially considered, many were rejected because of problems such as the difficulty in obtaining sufficient quantity with an acceptable level of purity and/or lack of clarity about the precise target in the kidney. Ultimately, the BNC selected cisplatin, gentamicin and N-phenylanthranilic acid as model compounds with well characterized nephrotoxic properties.

A fundamental component of the effort was the correlation of the test endpoints to the biological effects of interest using histopathology as the reference standard. Slides and histopathology data from all five HESI studies were initially reviewed by the BNC's Pathology Working Group to assess morphologic diagnoses and consistency in grading of finding severity, to identify key treatment-related findings for each toxicant, and to derive a common lexicon of morphologic diagnoses. Key agreements from this peer review were subsequently combined with the nascent kidney histopathology lexicon of the Critical

Path Institute (C-Path) Predictive Safety Testing Consortium Nephrotoxicity Working Group (PSTC NWG), and a unified renal histopathology lexicon was drafted following consensus between the HESI and C-Path PSTC NWG in October of 2006.

Biomarker Qualification: the Changing Landscape

As mentioned earlier, at the outset of this HESI program there was no process within regulatory agencies for review and approval of submitted biomarker qualification data. During the inception of the program, the participants' expectation was that it would progress via HESI's standard model of collaborative data development and evaluation across industry, academic, and government partners. It had been the BNC's original intention to work towards peer-reviewed publication of its results and conclusions and, ultimately, have the methodology validated by ICCVAM. A meeting of the HESI BNC in March 2006 modified this approach, as a representative of the FDA's Office of the Critical Path attended this meeting and described plans from within FDA to establish a new process for review of biomarker qualification data. Representatives of NIEHS were also present. In the proposed model, protocols and data could be submitted for review by the Pharm-Tox Coordinating Committee at FDA, although the process was in development and guidelines would be prepared later. At this session, a staff member from the National Toxicology Program Interagency Center for Evaluation of Alternative Toxicological Methods (NICEATM) offered support for the FDA proposal and indicated that ICCVAM focused more on method validation. A further update on the evolving FDA biomarker review process was presented to the HESI BNC in May 2007. As a consequence of this meeting HESI submitted a letter of intent to submit biomarker data to FDA for review and a qualification opinion.

The decision for the HESI BNC to follow a route of regulatory qualification was made only after extensive discussion, and of note, the HESI subcommittee had at the outset of the biomarker program considered whether HESI is an appropriate organization to undertake the identification and development of novel biomarkers (see point 5 in Table 15.2). HESI resolved that, while it was against its charter to engage in efforts to change regulatory policy, it was central to HESI's role to work with regulators to bring the best of science to bear to enable technically sound regulatory decisions. Nevertheless, it has to be acknowledged that the process of submission of a data package to the FDA (and, in parallel, the EMA) for review and decision did change the nature of the interaction on the BNC between regulators on the one hand and industry and academic representatives on the other. Many members of the BNC preferred the previous model where all participants, irrespective of affiliation, openly discussed the science and sought to arrive at a consensus interpretation of the data. In the period leading to the data submission, the regulatory members continued to participate in the BNC but, since they would eventually become the reviewers of the submitted data, they were required to be less forthcoming with opinions.

The preparation of the data for regulatory review and the subsequent rounds of questions and answers were protracted (Table 15.3) and labor intensive, for both the BNC

Table 15.3   HESI BIOMARKER QUALIFICATION Submission Timelines

- May 2008: Submitted qualification report to FDA/EMEA.
- July 2008: Meeting with FDA and EMA to discuss submission and first round of questions from the review by the qualifications teams of the two agencies.
- December 2008: Submitted formal written response and additional information per FDA-EMEA requests and queries.
- February 2009: Receipt of further comments and questions from FDA and EMA.
- April 2009: Document submitted as response to further questions from FDA-EMEA.
- September 2010: HESI received FDA qualification opinion.
- October 2010: EMA final qualification opinion published.

and the biomarker qualification teams at the agencies. Organizations participating on the committee during the submission process included: Allergan, Amgen, AstraZeneca, Bayer, Biogen-Idec, Biotrin, Bristol-Myers Squibb, GlaxoSmithKline, Johnson & Johnson, Merck, Pfizer, sanofi-aventis, Schering-Plough, Liverpool John Moores University, and the University of Arizona. Final qualification opinions were received from FDA and EMA [4,5] more than two years after the original data submission. It is evident from Table 15.3 that approximately 50% of the total review time was consumed by the time taken by the BNC to prepare written responses to the agency questions. This diverted the attention of the BNC from the previously agreed priority of publication in the open scientific literature. The postponement of the preparation of manuscripts was also influenced by a sense that it was appropriate to defer that activity until after the receipt of a regulatory review decision. It was only late in the review process that several manuscripts were prepared and finally published [6–8]. This delay was something which the BNC regretted and would recommend placing higher emphasis on peer review publication as a priority activity in the future.

It is now almost five years since the first qualification submission by the C-Path PSTC. For those who have participated in this process, it is clear that qualification of biomarkers is a complex and incremental process. To fully realize the potential of these markers for translational safety decision-making, many more data will be required to reinforce and enhance our understanding of the behavior of the qualified biomarkers (e.g., the temporal dynamic of their response during onset and recovery from chronic injury); to expand their use to additional animal species and humans and, where necessary, to provide additional biomarkers or define biomarker panels. To this end, the HESI BNC has generated additional data in rats which provide information on onset and recovery and the influence of gender. These data have been shared with the C-Path PSTC with a view to a joint HESI-PSTC supplementary qualification submission. The HESI BNC remains active but has decided to concentrate more on biomarker discovery (currently focused on miRNAs) and peer reviewed publication as an endpoint.

Ultimately, to show the value of the effort of assessing the utility of renal biomarkers, publications illustrating how qualified biomarkers have helped to enable initiation of clinical studies with compounds that presented with renal toxicity in pre-clinical evaluation is required. Although the regulatory aspects of qualification are important, such efforts should not derail or delay the development of scientifically robust data sets along with publication of the results. The availability of these important experiences will be key to sustaining meaningful activity in this area.

References

[1] Kramer JA, Pettit SD, Amin RP, Bertram TA, Car B, Cunningham M, et al. Overview of the application of transcription profiling using selected nephrotoxicants for toxicology assessment. Environ Health Perspect 2004;112:460–4.

[2] Amin RP, Vickers AE, Sistare F, Thompson KL, Roman RJ, Lawton M, et al. Identification of putative gene-based markers of renal toxicity. Environ Health Perspect 2004;112:465–79.

[3] Wallace KB, Hausner E, Herman E, Holt GD, MacGregor JT, Metz AL, et al. Serum troponins as biomarkers of drug-induced cardiac toxicity. Tox Path 2004;32:106–21.

[4] EMA. Qualification opinion ILSI/HESI submission of novel renal biomarkers for toxicity, In: http://www.emea.europa.eu/docs/en GB/document library/Regulatory and procedural guideline/2010/05/WC500090466.pdf. Accessed June 18, 2013.

[5] FDA. Non-clinical qualification of urinary biomarkers of nephrotoxicity: HESI nephrotoxicity qualification, In: http://www.fda.gov/Drugs/DevelopmentApprovalProcess/DrugDevelopmentTools QualificationProgram/ucm284076.htm; 2010. Accessed June 18, 2013.

[6] Harpur E, Ennulat D, Hoffman D, Betton G, Gautier J-C, Riefke B, et al. Biological qualification of biomarkers of nephrotoxicant-induced renal toxicity in two strains of male rat. Tox Sci 2011;122:235–52.

[7] Gautier JC, Riefke B, Walter J, Kurth P, Mylecraine L, Guilpin V, et al. Evaluation of novel biomarkers of nephrotoxicity in two strains of rat treated with Cisplatin. Toxicol Pathol 2010;38:943–56.

[8] Betton GR, Ennulat D, Hoffman D, Gautier J-C, Harpur E, Pettit S. Biomarkers of Collecting Duct Injury in Han-Wistar and Sprague-Dawley Rats Treated with N-Phenylanthranilic Acid. Toxicol Pathol 2012;40:682–94.

16

Vignette Regarding Consortia: C-Path Institute

Jeffrey Jacob

CANCER PREVENTION PHARMACEUTICALS AND CRITICAL PATH INSTITUTE, TUCSON, ARIZONA, USA

This is a vignette about biomarkers and about regulatory innovation. It is also about personal commitment and courage in FDA (Food and Drug Administration) champions and others who make change happen.

I was fortunate to be part of a founding group of people of the Critical Path Institute, which was inspired by the FDA's white paper describing the Critical Path initiative in 2005. We proposed an idea that we could create a neutral ground for industry, academic institutions, and government to work together in a precompetitive way to improve the process of medical product approval. This idea was only a working hypothesis at the time, yet the FDA actively supported it through the Genomics Group, the Office of Clinical Pharmacology and the Office of the Commissioner. Janet Woodcock, Felix Frueh, Federico Goodsaid, Wendy Sanhai, and other FDA scientists and clinicians actively worked in the early planning for what was to be called the C-Path Institute, and I worked directly with this FDA advocate group.

The C-Path Institute founding CEO, Raymond Woosley, provided the intellectual and management leadership for C-Path. He fostered a vision, and links with FDA management that opened an active, open and productive dialogue with the Agency. Through this dialogue, C-Path garnered input from FDA innovators, and drafted plans to create tangible and measurable efforts for regulatory innovation.

Ray Woosley recruited me as an engineer with a background in the commercialization of academic science, focusing on management of early stage drug development programs and investments in medical product development. I found every tool in my professional toolbox essential for the success of this effort, including curiosity, creativity, diplomacy, industry drug development know-how and deal making. For the first few months of its existence, the major operational activity for the C-Path Institute was the definition of 'what is most important to the FDA' and the cross-reference of this definition with pharmaceutical industry leaders to refine the C-Path focus. This initial assessment laid the groundwork for multiple consortia at C-Path.

The Predictive Safety Testing Consortium, or PSTC, was the first of several consortia at C-Path. PSTC served as the model for all subsequent C-Path consortia. Although some of the initiatives didn't evolve beyond their planning stages, they all taught us what we needed to know for the success of the PSTC. The PSTC has proved to be one of the most

The Path from Biomarker Discovery to Regulatory Qualification. http://dx.doi.org/10.1016/B978-0-12-391496-5.00016-8

successful initiatives linked to the Critical Path at the FDA and is continually cited by FDA and Industry leaders as a model for public/private collaboration. It has also informed more recent European initiatives such as the Innovative Medicines Initiative (IMI).

Why did PSTC succeed? In my view, the unique alignment between the FDA and industry was the critical element in the success of the PSTC. The PSTC was led by pharmaceutical industry scientists, and clinicians with technical expertise and a personal commitment to change the regulatory application of biomarkers. The initial driving force included Novartis (Jacky Vonderscher), Merck (Frank Sistare) and Pfizer (Denise Robinson-Gravatt), but these companies were quickly joined by over a dozen others, such that *all* of the PSTC Executive Committee contributed in the early work of the PSTC. For the initial Working Group, Novartis volunteered their previous work in the development of nephrotoxicity biomarkers as part of a CRADA with the FDA, and Merck contributed a large body of internal research results.

As a first cause, eight pharmaceutical companies agreed to collaborate in the areas of biomarkers of nephrotoxicity, hepatotoxicity, carcinogenicity, and muscle toxicity. Once verbal agreement was obtained from these companies, the next challenge was the creation of an acceptable legal framework. The complex organization of these companies, and the multilateral negotiations required, dictated that over a year was needed to complete the legal collaboration agreement.

C-Path provided a neutral and unique framework for this collaboration, such that PSTC could uniquely address intellectual property issues and proposals for regulatory change. This set the PSTC apart from the organization of other collaborative efforts such as ILSI and PhRMA. The legal agreement for the PSTC was its greatest organizational challenge – and perhaps its greatest accomplishment. It created acceptable concepts for handling intellectual property, dealing with anti-trust concerns, and for managing the consortium through a C-Path leadership team.

Anti-trust concerns reflected both real issues as well as perceived ones, and proved to be difficult to overcome. A breakthrough in drafting the anti-trust language happened at a working dinner C-Path hosted in Washington DC. Company representatives provided general support for this language, but many were reluctant to push their company lawyers and management. Janet Woodcock, CDER Center Director, participated in this meeting and directly told the PSTC team that the appropriate anti-trust language HAD to be found, because the PSTC HAD to succeed. This emphatic support enabled each representative to return to his or her corresponding company and effectively persuade their lawyers to collectively discuss the anti-trust statement. At the defining conference call there were twenty lawyers on the line. All but one company in the consortium agreed with the proposed language.

Eventually, sixteen companies joined the PSTC and each of the working groups began its effort to qualify biomarkers for drug development. Working groups were set up to propose and qualify biomarkers for hepatotoxicity, renal toxicity, carcinogenicity, and muscle toxicity. An executive committee was set up to oversee all projects and maintain the support needed within each company. Each company would propose biomarkers they had been working on internally, and share data from internally conducted studies. As these were biomarkers of preclinical drug safety evaluation, a scientist with extensive experience in this field (William Mattes) was recruited to lead the PSTC as Director.

The kidney biomarker panel originally proposed by Novartis and Merck led to a new biomarker qualification process and documented 'qualification approval letters' from the FDA, the EMA (European Medicines Agency) and the PMDA (the Pharmaceuticals and Medical Devices Agency, Japan). It also led to hope that there could be a new type of cooperation to advance regulatory science – both by contribution of proprietary science from the industry and 'outside the box' thinking by the FDA. The final outcome of this effort is still yet to be seen, but C-Path and others are currently working on scores of potential biomarker qualification programs both in the US and with other regulatory agencies throughout the world. It should be possible to apply this model for the translation of other scientific innovations into modernized regulatory policy.

Being part of this evolution was extremely rewarding and educational for me personally. I made many new professional friends and was reminded once again that sometimes, timing – as well as strong will from talented and well placed people – is very important. Although others are in the business of bringing companies together to advance science, C-Path was (and continues to be) in the right place at the right time to translate the science directly into regulatory innovations. An essential learning was that projects needed to be suggested by the FDA, agreed to by the industry, to have champions from both venues, and to have some immediate applications that could be pushed ahead relatively quickly into regulatory innovation. In this case, vision and courage needed to go together, because the vision behind these difficult changes often exacted a high career cost. Nonetheless, a new Biomarker Qualification Process emerged from this link between vision and courage at the FDA, the pharmaceutical industry and the leaders and members of the PSTC.

17

The Telemetric and Holter ECG Warehouse to Enable the Validation and Development of Novel Electrocardiographic Markers

Jean-Philippe Couderc

UNIVERSITY OF ROCHESTER MEDICAL SCHOOL, ROCHESTER, NEW YORK, USA

Introduction

Biomarkers are associated with slightly different definitions depending on the context in which they are used. For instance, in regulatory environments biomarkers are defined as 'laboratory measurement that reflects the activity of a disease process' [1], while in the clinical world the biomarkers are tools 'to identify high risk individuals, to diagnose a disease condition promptly and accurately, and to effectively prognosticate and treat patients with disease', while in molecular biology research they are generally described as 'cellular, biomechanical or molecular alterations that are measurable in biological media such as human tissues, cells, or fluids'. In this section, we will consider the broader definition released by the National Institutes of Health: 'a characteristic that is objectively measured and evaluated as an indicator of normal biologic processes, pathogenic processes, or pharmacologic responses to a therapeutic intervention'. We will refer in the following to electrocardiographic markers rather than electrocardiographic biomarkers, keeping in mind this latest and broader definition.

In this vignette, we aim to describe the development of an initiative initially linked to one specific marker: the QT interval. We initiated the Telemetric and Holter ECG Warehouse (THEW) following considerable interest, expressed by numerous parties, in better understanding and improving this electrocardiographic marker. We will describe the inception of this initiative, hoping the readers will benefit from our experience. Over the years, our consortium has grown into a platform sustaining a large spectrum of activities. All of these activities have one common denominator which is at the core of our mission: the science of quantitative electrocardiography [2]. Quantitative electrocardiography is the field of extracting information from the body surface electrocardiogram (ECG) that is relevant to the diagnosis or/and the treatment of patients.

The Path from Biomarker Discovery to Regulatory Qualification. http://dx.doi.org/10.1016/B978-0-12-391496-5.00017-X

Electrocardiography will soon celebrate its 110th year of existence. In 1903, the 43-year-old Dutch physician and physiologist Willen Einthoven (1860–1927) released a publication describing the first electrocardiogram. While the five normal inflections (P, Q, R, T) he initially described remain routinely used by cardiologists and other health professionals, the recording technologies have evolved profoundly. Undoubtedly, the most important technological advance in modern electrocardiography has been the use of ECG recording in an electronic format. The inception of digital electrocardiography led to major improvement: 1) increasing the length of the ECG recordings, 2) increasing its precision, 3) miniaturizing the recording devices, and 4) developing hybrid technologies such as the implantable recorders and other ambulatory apparatuses. Electrocardiographic tools are sometimes perceived as old, lackadaisical technologies compared to medical imaging such as 3D echocardiography and to magnetic resonance imaging tools. Yet, one would note that ECGs have remained one of the most commonly used investigational tools in clinics and clinical drug safety studies. The reasons are manifold: it is an easily accessible technology, it is a cost-efficient tool, and it is the only non-invasive tool currently available that can gain direct insights into the electrical state of the heart.

In the following, we will describe how the idea of our consortium started following discussions amongst federal regulators; how its development was attractive to the National Institutes of Health, and finally how we developed a large scientific network gathering worldwide organizations. The first part of this chapter describes how a set of blockbuster drugs led to important changes in the evaluation of new drugs by the Food and Drug Administration (FDA), and the development of ECG-specific safety studies (thorough QT studies), and finally, how numerous improvements and the genesis of a 'biomarker' were triggered during this process. In the second part, we will describe the creation of our consortium and its development, the discussions with FDA regulators, and the submission of novel biomarkers to the Agency.

QT Interval as a Safety Marker in Drug Development

The safety of commercial drugs related to QT/QTc prolongation was raised at the end of the nineties following the market withdrawal of a couple of drugs due to their cardiotoxicity (Astemizole and Grepafloxacin in 1999, Cisapride in 2000) [3]. Thereafter, the increased vigilance of the Food and Drug Administration (FDA) and the pharmaceutical companies led to the finding that this issue was present in a large spectrum of drug families, including opioids, antimigraine, antimalarial, anti-asthmatic, antihistamines, anti-infectives, antineoplatics, antilipemic, diuretics, gastrointestinal, hormones, antidepressants and antipsychotics. Most non-cardiac QT-prolonging drugs have a direct blocking effect on the rapid component of the delayed repolarization potassium current (I_{kr}), and predispose patients to a specific type of polymorphic ventricular arrhythmia called 'torsades de pointes' (TdPs). An exhaustive list of the drugs that prolong the QT/QTc interval, and thus carry risk for triggering TdPs is provided at www.qtdrugs.org. [05-06-2013]. Only a limited number of cases of TdPs were reported amongst the millions of patients taking these drugs, but pharmaceutical companies and regulators were challenged to design an approach to identify these compounds within the framework of the new drug application process.

QT Interval: from a Biomarker to a Surrogate Marker

The drug safety issue around QTc prolongation has considerably impacted the development and evaluation of new drugs for pharmaceutical companies, and it has stimulated research, technologies and businesses, not without some uncertainty from the various stakeholders. Importantly, the QTc interval was rapidly accepted as a drug safety marker because of multiple scientific reports which demonstrated its association with the occurrence of life-threatening arrhythmias in a broad context of use.

The congenital long QT syndrome (LQTS) is probably the most relevant example. The LQTS is an inherited disease caused by genetic defects in transmembrane ion channel subunit that may be linked to 2 to 5% of the 300,000 yearly sudden cardiac deaths in the US. These patients are at high risk for cardiac death due to the development of ventricular tachycardia (and TdPs) degenerating in ventricular fibrillation [4–6]. Typically, the arrhythmias occur in conjunction with vigorous physical exercise and emotional stress. Among numerous mutations identified in the seven LQTS genes, LQT1 and LQT2 (HERG, KCNH2) represent the majority of cases (88%) whereas LQT3 accounts only for 7% and the others are very rare. The protein encoded by the HERG (KCNH2) subunit serves the I_{Kr} current [7]. A mutation in this gene has been associated with a reduction (partial blockade) of the I_{Kr} current leading to the phenotypic ECG representation known in LQT2 patients [8].

In a prospective longitudinal study of 328 families with the LQTS, it was shown that for every 10 msec increase in QTc duration there was a 5% exponential increase of the risk of cardiac events [5]. In a study of LQTS family members from the International LQTS Registry, the hazard ratio for cardiac events by QTc duration were 1.43 for QTc between 0.45 s and 0.46 s, 2.42 for QTc between 0.47 s and 0.50 s and 4.84 for QTc > 0.50 s, when compared to QTc ≤ 0.44 s [9] (Fig. 17.1).

The mechanistic link between the hereditary and the acquired form of the LQTS was identified in several publications released between 1993 and 1997. The first relevant work was reported by Woosley et al. [10]. This group described the cardiotoxic mechanisms of terfenadine blocking the I_{Kr} current in the feline ventricular myocyte at therapeutically relevant concentrations. Two years later, Sanguinetti et al. reported that the locus of the most prevalent form of the congenital LQTS (LQT2) was the HERG (KCNH2) gene that expressed the same I_{Kr} current in xenopus oocytes [7]. The concept of HERG being a primary human ventricular target for other non-cardiac drugs with QT liability was confirmed with cisapride [11]. Finally, numerous drugs subsequently showed similar findings [12,13].

The definition of the QT interval is concise and clear. It is a time interval starting from the beginning of the QRS complex (the earliest from all available ECG leads) and ending at the offset of the T-wave (lead specific QT interval are usually reported or the longest interval from all available leads). The QT interval represents the duration of

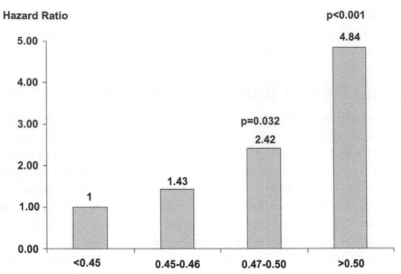

FIGURE 17.1 Evolution of the hazard ratios for cardiac events in relation to the QTc interval duration in the long QT syndrome. Figure from reference 9.

the ventricular repolarization process of the heart ventricles. If the prolongation of the QT interval strongly predisposes individuals to cardiac arrhythmias, this marker suffers from strong weaknesses which include a weak link between experimental and clinical events (specifically in drug evaluation), and the lack of standardization in measurement methods [3,14]. Indeed, multiple factors affect the QT intervals including:

1) physiological factors such as gender, heart rate and autonomic regulation, and
2) technical factors such as lead selection, ECG signal specifications, and T-wave offset identification.

The role of gender is important when investigating the relationship between QT prolongation and cardiac events. Women are more prone to develop TdP than men during the administration of medicines which have the potential to block the I_{Kr} current. Women have a slightly longer QT interval duration, but also present specific T-wave morphology on the surface ECGs [15–17]. It is believed that testosterone can play an important role in modulating cardiac repolarization, and that it plays a protective role by shortening the QT interval [18]. In addition to gender differences, there is a large heterogeneity of responses from patients exposed to drugs modifying the intra-cellular potassium currents. This emphasizes the role of patient predisposition to QT prolongation. The effect of a repolarization-prolonging drug may be modulated by various factors such as the subject's repolarization reserve, the subject's genetic make-up or the presence of an asymptomatic LQTS mutation. Such patients have a reduced repolarization reserve which makes them more susceptible to potassium blocking agent [19]. The penetrance of this type of clinically silent abnormal repolarization state is unknown but it is believed to be significant in the general population. In other subjects, the drug-induced ion dysfunction becomes malignant because of the presence of a drug interaction. Most QT-prolonging drugs that have only a small effect on the I_{Kr} ion current may lead to significant QT prolongation when administrated with other drugs affecting drug metabolism (e.g., through their effect on the cytochrome P-450 enzymatic system) [20]. Thus, the identification of individuals with an acquired or induced predisposition to QT prolongation is a significant issue. The role of heart rate and autonomic regulation will be discussed later, since they remain a very vivid field of research in which our consortium is very active.

The technical factors influencing the measurement of the QT interval are multiple and we will describe their associated challenges and how they have been addressed in the next section. Importantly, the identification of the end of the T-wave which indicates the end of the QT interval is not based on any standard measurement approach and thereby is qualified on its precision rather than its accuracy, which has impacted profoundly the way QT measurements are done in drug safety studies.

The Thorough QT Studies (TQT)

The regulatory response to the challenge of assessing drug safety related to QTc prolongation was released in collaboration with the International Conference for Harmonization (ICH) in a guidance document (E14). The document recommended the implementation of safety assessment studies specifically designed to evaluate the potential of new compounds to prolong the QT interval (and usually conducted prior to Phase III development). Readers are referred to the description by B. Darpo for more information about TQT studies [21]. However, while the E14 document was being developed, the FDA made a public appeal for the development of both a centralized warehouse for hosting standard 12-lead ECGs acquired in TQT studies, and a standard format to store these signals. The so-called aECG format, 'a' (standing for 'annotated'), was created following the Health Level 7 (HL7) Regulated Clinical Research Information Management, which is a working group to enhance information management during pre-clinical research, clinical research and regulatory evaluation of therapeutic products and procedure. The aECG standard format was accepted by the American National Standards Institute in 2004. The warehouse was built by Mortara Instruments (Milwaukee, WI) and it is widely used by pharmaceutical companies and other contract research organizations to submit their ECG data from TQT studies to the FDA for review.

Unfortunately, from the point of view of ECG marker development, this initiative was disappointing, perhaps because its development was not primarily driven by the search for improved science and technologies, but rather to deliver a technical platform to facilitate the submission of ECG signals and metrics to regulatory bodies. Despite these limitations, the FDA and the Cardiac Safety Research Consortium succeeded in developing a database of standard 12-lead ECGs (containing data from baseline and the positive arms of TQT studies) designed for the validation and test of QT measurement algorithms. This database was carefully crafted to optimize the validation of QT measurement algorithms [22]. Its limitation is that pharmaceutical companies do not really have strong incentives to submit data from compounds with positive QT signals (apart from the positive control arm).

As we will see in the next section, a lot of research work around QT as a surrogate marker of TdPs was triggered by the regulatory concern of drug safety. It led to a significant improvement in the ability of computers to measure and monitor the QT interval [14].

Improving the QT Marker

During this initial period, the regulatory interest in assessing drug-induced QT prolongation became a significant driving force, not only for developing research to better understand the effect of drugs and their concentrations on the QT interval, but also to control the various factors known to have an effect on the duration of the QT intervals, such as heart rate and the autonomic regulation of the heart. Thus, the regulatory interest led to a strong effort in scientific research, which is reflected in Fig. 17.2 describing the throughput of scientific literature (number of publications) related to QT interval and drug. These publications encompass works on the improvement of QT measurement, and a better understanding of the effect of drugs on the QT interval following (effect of heart rate, gender, drug concentration, study designs, amongst many others). We will briefly

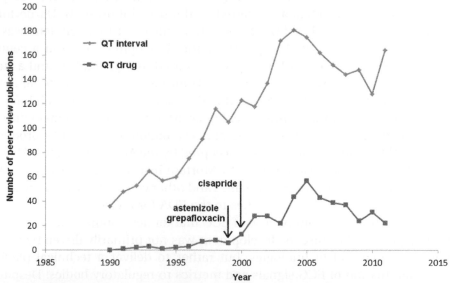

FIGURE 17.2 Number of scientific peer-review publications released by year between 1990 and 2011. The search was based on two keywords: 'QT interval' and 'QT drugs' entered into Google Scholar search engine. It is noteworthy that the regulatory interest itself has been an effective trigger of research contributing to increase our understanding of strengths and weakness of QT prolongation as a drug safety marker. The vertical arrows mark the time of market withdrawal of the labeled drugs.

discuss the factors that led to the inception of our initiative, i.e., the need to better evaluate the role of physiological confounding factors including, but not limited to, the effect of heart rate, signal quality and autonomic regulation on the QT intervals.

The level of precision required for QT measurements in TQT studies is higher than that expected in standard ECG equipment (designed primarily for clinical use). In clinical settings, a QT interval longer than 440 msec is considered prolonged, between 450 and 470 ms is borderline, and values greater than 470 msec raise concern. The QT interval is strongly abnormal when it equals or is greater than 500 msec. The focus in clinics has always been the accuracy of QT measurements and the detection of LQTS, and, as described in the study by Viskin et al., most physicians cannot identify the presence of an LQTS because they either do not measure QT interval well or they do not calculate the heart rate correction properly [23].

In drug safety studies, investigators have been looking for drug effects of the order of 5–10 msec, and only trained personnel could ensure a level of precision good enough to detect such a signal in a study with an acceptable number of individuals ($N > 50$). The challenge of precise QT measurement was associated with a cost that was driven by the number of individuals to enroll, the analytics, and the manual QT interval measurement on thousands of ECG tracing acquired during the TQT studies. This created strong incentives to improve the QT measurements; i.e., to increase its precision in order to decrease the size of the TQT studies. This was highlighted in the special issue of the Annals of Non-invasive Electrocardiology in which we invited companies to present their method (or improved method) for QT measurements [14]. Most of these publications relied on a set of ECG recordings from TQT studies shared by pharmaceutical companies. Importantly, all methods were able to detect the positive control signal induced by moxifloxacin (usual positive control substance for QT prolongation used in TQT). However, it became difficult to compare the precision of these methods, since they were based on different studies with different levels of quality and design (gender and age distributions, etc.).

QT, Heart Rate and Autonomic Regulation

The issue related to the relationship between heart rate and QT interval duration has been widely published [24–27], yet it remains a significant challenge in studies involving compounds which have a direct effect on heart rate. Obviously, the issue is linked to the potential contamination of the QT measurements by heart rate changes driven by drug effects.

The relationship of QT to the RR interval is complex. It is primarily influenced by the autonomic regulation of the heart [28]. Modeling the QT/RR relationships, so-called QT-RR dynamicity, from continuous Holter recordings, was studied in healthy subjects in LQTS patients [29], and various cardiac populations where it found potential clinical value [30]. QT-RR dynamicity is, unfortunately, a crude method for characterizing the relationship between QT and preceding RR intervals. Firstly, it neglects the effect of RR history by relying on the immediately preceding RR interval, or it linearizes it by using the mean values of previous RR intervals. Secondly, it merges the QT response to acceleration and deceleration of heart rate which has been shown to be different [31]. Alternative approaches using modeling of the QT-RR coupling have been suggested [32,33]. These show that:

1) the QT interval is influenced by the history of RR intervals from the preceding 2 minutes, and
2) the influence of the most distant RR intervals is small in comparison to the most recent ones.

To address the problem of QT dependency to heart rate, other creative solutions have been proposed, such as the RR bin method [34] and the beat-to-beat QT method [35], which are amongst the most published. The purpose of this section is not to describe in detail these techniques but rather to highlight how the development of technologies related to drug safety relies on the availability of relevant data. Indeed, as of today, there is a set of creative technical solutions proposed to address this issue, yet the identification of the 'best' method(s) remains elusive because of the lack of data from studies investigating drugs that impact the heart rate. This has slowed down our advances in this field. Importantly, the common denominator of all these approaches is to rely on continuous ECG recordings in order to gather a wealth of information that can vary across techniques such as a large series of QT-RR couplets acquired in individuals on and off drugs.

Inception of the Telemetric and Holter ECG Warehouse (THEW): a Model to Develop Academia-Regulators-Industries Partnerships

The Telemetric and Holter ECG Warehouse, so-called THEW, is an initiative started in 2005 after an unofficial discussion between regulators from the Center for Drug Evaluation and Research at the FDA, academic individuals and individuals from contract research organizations. Interestingly, this discussion did not take place at an FDA campus, but in a rental car in Milwaukee while driving back to the airport from a seminar organized by an ECG equipment company. During this seminar, vivid discussions highlighted the limitation of the measurements of the QT/QTc interval from standard 12-lead ECGs due to the lack of information related to previous history of heart rate. This discussion actively continued, diverging from the need to better assess the role of heart rate, to improving the assessment of the role of the autonomic regulation, to the dynamic features of the QT interval. During this discussion, it became quite obvious that access to continuous ECG recordings was the key to improving the necessary understanding and the development of novel ECG markers that could complement QT interval prolongation.

The idea of developing a digital repository for continuous ECGs did not sound very challenging technically, since our ECG Core Laboratory at the Heart Research Follow-up Program in Rochester (NY) already hosted a large database of continuous and Holter

ECGs from clinical trials such as the DEFINITE [36], OAT [37] and MADIT trials [38,39]. Rather, the challenge was to align activities around such a consortium to gather all stakeholders on a common platform.

This discussion made it obvious that, even if Holter ECGs from TQT studies were not reviewed by the regulators, there was a common interest in analyzing continuous ECGs recorded in these studies, and from such a task, many opportunities to develop new ECG markers were very likely to appear. This initiative would be aligned with the strategies of the FDA to improve tools and technologies in drug evaluation as described in the Critical Path Initiative report.[1] So, the timing was right. This problem was not limited to human data, but also existed in the pre-clinical world. As an example, pre-clinical tools were suffering from a lack of automation to analyze the electrical activity of animals exposed to these new compounds.

The availability of a warehouse which gathered thousands of human recordings seemed to be welcomed by all players: regulators, US and European corporations, as well as academic institutions. This was a crucial point. Indeed, the development of an animal branch of the THEW did not meet this common interest. And, not surprisingly, the goal to develop an animal branch for the THEW failed due to lack of incentive from multiple stakeholders.

Involving the FDA and Industry

The THEW concept was welcomed by the FDA. We obtained full support through the signature of a private–public partnership.[2] The signing of this agreement was accompanied by a series of meetings at the FDA campus, to which individuals from pharmaceutical companies and ECG equipment companies were invited. The first meeting occurred in January 2008 and the second in April 2009. We opted to develop a donation program to ensure that seed funds would be available to build the initial THEW infrastructure. Five companies all present at this meeting agreed to contribute. The core IT infrastructure of the warehouse was developed and ready to host large amounts of data at the beginning of 2009. The next challenge was to convince different companies to share their data. Initially, many companies refused to do so. It took much effort and discussion between lawyers from different stakeholders to finally agree on a Data Sharing Agreement (DSA). The DSA defined a precise legal framework for the transfer of data ownership, to protect the former data owner as well as the individuals from whom the data were acquired. A couple of months after its release, the THEW DSAs were signed by two major pharmaceutical companies and ECG signals from TQT studies started flowing into the repository.

Less than one year after discussion of the THEW with the regulators, we had built a repository hosting the largest publicly available set of full 24 hour digital Holter

---

[1]http://www.fda.gov/ScienceResearch/SpecialTopics/CriticalPathInitiative/default.htm [06-07-2013].
[2]http://www.fda.gov/AboutFDA/PartnershipsCollaborations/PublicPrivatePartnershipProgram/ucm231128.htm [06-08-2013].

recordings in the world. We worked on adding several databases from our own institution, including those from large cohorts of healthy individuals. We then further developed the database by submitting a R24 grant proposal to the National Heart Lung and Blood Institute (NHLBI).

Participation by the National Institutes of Health

The challenges of developing a scientific resource in an academic setting are two-fold: relevant scientific productivity and financial sustainability. The first one depends on the quality and scientific credibility of the data resource, while financial sustainability requires designing a mechanism to generate income while fitting the legal requirements of not-for-profit organization such as our University. Consequently, our first step was to seek NIH support through the R24 program. This program is designed to help scientists develop resources to service the worldwide scientific community. Of course, as with any NIH program, these funds are time-limited, so the NIH proposes the so-called 'program income' mechanism[3] enabling principal investigators to develop a simple 'business' model in which to access users' fees. This money is then used to sustain or further develop the resources. It is noteworthy that we were careful to emphasize our intent to use the NIH funds to improve drug safety and not to develop technologies to decrease drug development costs. In the NIH proposal, we planned to fill the scientific gaps by developing a platform in which all stakeholders could consider the use of a publicly available database.

The grant project was presented to the Institute in October 2008 as a prerequisite for the application to this resource program. The concept was simply to expand the warehouse. The access would be free for academia, and would be purchased by for-profit organizations to support the cost of maintaining the initiative. The membership would provide full rights to these companies to develop their own technologies for using the data and gaining intellectual property from their work without any strings attached by our initiative. This last detail has been crucial to the development of the THEW, because it has retained the incentives needed for corporate participation. The letter of intent for applying to the R24 program at the NHLBI was sent in September 2008. In March 2009 the proposal was granted a multi-million dollar award that has supported our activities until today [05-06-2013].

Facilitating the Submission of New ECG Markers to the FDA

One of the outcomes of the collaboration between the member organizations of THEW has been the 'Electrocardiographic Marker(s) Submission Form to The Office of

---

[3]http://grants.nih.gov/grants/policy/nihgps_2003/nihgps_part8.htm

Translational Science (OTS) of the Center for Drug Evaluation and Research, FDA'. A THEW working group was formed which gathered scientists from the FDA, academia and industry. The objective of the group was to facilitate the submission of novel ECG markers for drug safety to the Agency.

First, we defined an ECG marker as:

> *'A characteristic of the electrocardiographic signal measured from the body surface that is objectively measured and evaluated as an indicator of normal electrophysiological processes, pathogenic processes, or pharmacologic responses to a xenobiotic exposure.'*

ECG markers are used in clinical practice to identify risk of disease, to diagnose disease and its severity, to guide intervention strategies and to monitor patient responses to therapy. ECG markers may predict whether a drug or other intervention is safe and effective in a shorter time and at lower cost than clinical outcomes studies.

A form was designed in order to provide preliminary information to the OTS to trigger the process of internal review. In the list of information included were the following points:

1) The context of use, which could be individual-based marker, population-based marker, diagnosis, prognosis, or assessment of response to intervention.
2) The description of the supporting data available at the time of the submission: animal, *in vitro*, or clinical studies could be considered.
3) A description of the current validation work (including the use of database from the THEW if available).
4) The list of related publications supporting the qualification of the proposed marker(s).

The submission form is available for download on the THEW website, and is accepted by the Agency for initiating any submission. In order to maintain the confidentiality of future submissions, our initiative is not involved in the follow-up of submissions based on the form.

Currently, the development and validation of QT measurements represents a small part of the research activities conducted using the data from the THEW [40–42]. The development of novel ECG markers or techniques to improve QT induced by drugs has shifted toward new methods to measure dynamic aspects of the QT intervals [42,43] and novel ECG markers for drug safety [43–47].

Conclusions and Perspectives

Currently, the THEW initiative gathers members from 38 academic and not-for-profit organizations located in five continents; Asia, North America, South America, Europe and Australia. The total number of peer review publications based on THEW data was 22 in December 2010. A total of 16 companies have become members since the start of its membership program. These include corporations such as Philips Healthcare and Samsung Electronics, which are currently working on the data from our repository. Technologies that have been developed and validated on data from the THEW are used today by various companies, not only in the drug safety arena but also in equipment marketed in Europe and in the United States. Importantly, several organizations have developed and validated their QT measurement techniques based on data from THEW[4].

In conclusion, the incentive to gather efforts such as the THEW depends on the existence of gaps between deliverables of private organizations and the expectations of regulatory agencies. The ability to generate fruitful consortia is correlated with the ability to create working synergies between the various players and by defining the right value proposition to the stakeholders. In the case of THEW, both the weakness and the uniqueness of the QT interval as an ECG marker have played a crucial role in gathering stakeholders and resources to develop the initiative. It has also matured into an international effort with broader development and scientific activities than initially planned.

References

[1] Katz R. Biomarkers and surrogate markers: an FDA perspective. NeuroRx 2004;1:189–95.

[2] Couderc JP. The telemetric and holter ECG warehouse initiative (THEW): A data repository for the design, implementation and validation of ECG-related technologies. Engineering in Medicine and Biology Society (EMBC), 2010 Annual International Conference of the IEEE 2010:6252–5.

[3] Whellan DJ, Green CL, Piccini JP, Krucoff MW. QT as a safety biomarker in drug development. Clin Pharmacol Ther 2009;86:101–4.

[4] Keating M, Atkinson D, Dunn C, Timothy K, Vincent GM, Leppert M. Linkage of a cardiac arrhythmia, the long QT syndrome, and the Harvey ras-1 gene. Science 1991;252:704–6.

[5] Moss AJ, Schwartz PJ, Crampton RS, Tzivoni D, Locati EH, MacCluer J, et al. The long QT syndrome. Prospective longitudinal study of 328 families. Circulation 1991;84:1136–44. Ref Type: Journal.

[6] Zareba W, Moss AJ, le Cessie S, Locati EH, Robinson JL, Hall WJ, et al. Risk of cardiac events in family members of patients with long QT syndrome. J Am Coll Cardiol 1995;26:1685–91.

[7] Sanguinetti MC, Curran ME, Spector PS, Keating MT. Spectrum of HERG K+-channel dysfunction in an inherited cardiac arrhythmia. Proc Natl Acad Sci U S A 1996;93:2208–12.

[8] Moss AJ, Zareba W, Benhorin J, Locati EH, Hall WJ, Robinson JL, et al. ECG T-wave patterns in genetically distinct forms of the hereditary long QT syndrome. Circulation 1995;92:2929–34.

[9] Zareba W, Moss AJ, le CS, Locati EH, Robinson JL, Hall WJ, et al. Risk of cardiac events in family members of patients with long QT syndrome. J Am Coll Cardiol 1995;26:1685–91.

[10] Woosley RL, Chen Y, Freiman JP, Gillis RA. Mechanism of the cardiotoxic actions of terfenadine. JAMA 1993;269:1532–6.

[11] Rampe D, Roy ML, Dennis A, Brown AM. A mechanism for the proarrhythmic effects of cisapride (Propulsid): high affinity blockade of the human cardiac potassium channel HERG. FEBS Lett 1997; 417:28–32.

---

[4]http://thew-project.org/Publication_main.html

[12] De PF, Poluzzi E, Cavalli A, Recanatini M, Montanaro N. Safety of non-antiarrhythmic drugs that prolong the QT interval or induce torsade de pointes: an overview. Drug Saf 2002;25:263–86.

[13] Rampe D, Murawsky MK. Blockade of the human cardiac K+ channel Kv1.5 by the antibiotic erythromycin. Naunyn Schmiedebergs Arch Pharmacol 1997;355:743–50.

[14] Couderc JP, Zareba W. An update on QT measurement and interpretation methodologies. Ann Noninvasive Electrocardiol 2009;14(Suppl. 1):S1–2.

[15] Bidoggia H, Maciel JP, Capalozza N, Mosca S, Blaksley EJ, Valverde E, et al. Sex-dependent electrocardiographic pattern of cardiac repolarization. Am Heart J 2000;140:430–6.

[16] Lehmann MH, Yang H. Sexual dimorphism in the electrocardiographic dynamics of human ventricular repolarization: characterization in true time domain. Circulation 2001;104:32–8.

[17] Rautaharju PM, Zhou SH, Wong S, Calhoun HP, Berenson GS, Prineas R, et al. Sex differences in the evolution of the electrocardiographic QT interval with age. Can J Cardiol 1992;8:690–5.

[18] Bidoggia H, Maciel JP, Capalozza N, Mosca S, Blaksley EJ, Valverde E, et al. Sex differences on the electrocardiographic pattern of cardiac repolarization: possible role of testosterone. Am Heart J 2000;140:678–83.

[19] Napolitano C, Schwartz PJ, Brown AM, Ronchetti E, Bianchi L, Pinnavaia A, et al. Evidence for a cardiac ion channel mutation underlying drug-induced QT prolongation and life-threatening arrhythmias. J Cardiovasc Electrophysiol 2000;11:691–6.

[20] Desta Z, Soukhova N, Mahal SK, Flockhart DA. Interaction of cisapride with the human cytochrome P450 system: metabolism and inhibition studies. Drug Metab Dispos 2000;28:789–800.

[21] Darpo B. The thorough QT/QTc study 4 years after the implementation of the ICH E14 guidance. Br J Pharmacol 2010;159:49–57.

[22] Kligfield P, Green CL, Mortara J, Sager P, Stockbridge N, Li M, et al. The Cardiac Safety Research Consortium electrocardiogram warehouse: thorough QT database specifications and principles of use for algorithm development and testing. Am Heart J 2010;160:1023–8.

[23] Viskin S, Rosovski U, Sands AJ, Chen E, Kistler PM, Kalman JM, et al. Inaccurate electrocardiographic interpretation of long QT: the majority of physicians cannot recognize a long QT when they see one. Heart Rhythm 2005;2:569–74.

[24] Couderc JP, Xiaojuan X, Zareba W, Moss AJ. Assessment of the Stability of the Individual-Based Correction of QT Interval for Heart Rate. Ann Noninvasive Electrocardiol 2005;10:25–34.

[25] Extramiana F, Maison-Blanche P, Badilini F, Beaufils P, Leenhardt A. Individual QT-R-R relationship: average stability over time does not rule out an individual residual variability: implication for the assessment of drug effect on the QT interval. Ann Noninvasive Electrocardiol 2005;10:169–78.

[26] Malik M. Problems of heart rate correction in assessment of drug-induced QT interval prolongation. J Cardiovasc Electrophysiol 2001;12:411–20.

[27] Malik M, Farbom P, Batchvarov V, Hnatkova K, Camm AJ. Relation between QT and RR intervals is highly individual among healthy subjects: implications for heart rate correction of the QT interval. Heart 2002;87:220–8.

[28] Coumel P, Maison-Blanche P. QT dynamicity as a predictor for arrhythmia development. In: Ota A, Breithardt C, editors. Myocardial repolarization: from gene to bedside. NY: Futura publishing; 2001.

[29] Neyroud N, Maison-Blanche P, Denjoy I, Chevret S, Donger C, Dausse E, et al. Diagnostic performance of QT interval variables from 24 h electrocardiography in the long QT syndrome. Eur Heart J 1998;19:158–65.

[30] Chevalier P, Burri H, Adeleine P, Kirkorian G, Lopez M, Leizorovicz A, et al. QT dynamicity and sudden death after myocardial infarction: results of a long-term follow-up study. J Cardiovasc Electrophysiol 2003;14:227–33.

[31] Franz MR, Swerdlow CD, Liem LB, Schaefer J. Cycle length dependence of human action potential duration *in vivo*. Effects of single extrastimuli, sudden sustained rate acceleration and deceleration, and different steady-state frequencies. J Clin Invest 1988;82:972–9.

[32] Pueyo E, Smetana P, Laguna P, Malik M. Estimation of the QT/RR hysteresis lag. J Electrocardiol 2003;36(Suppl.):187–90.

[33] Halamek J, Jurak P, Villa M, Soucek M, Frana P, Nykodym J, et al. Dynamic coupling between heart rate and ventricular repolarisation. Biomed Tech (Berl) 2007;52:255–63.

[34] Badilini F, Maison-Blanche P, Childers R, Coumel P. QT interval analysis on ambulatory electro-cardiogram recordings: a selective beat averaging approach. Med Biol Eng Comput 1999;37:71–9.

[35] Fossa AA, Langdon G, Couderc JP, Zhou M, Darpo B, Wilson F, et al. The Use of Beat-to-Beat Electrocardiogram Analysis to Distinguish QT/QTc Interval Changes Caused by Moxifloxacin From Those Caused by Vardenafil. Clin Pharmacol Ther 2011;90:449–54.

[36] Kadish A, Dyer A, Daubert JP, Quigg R, Estes NA, Anderson KP, et al. Prophylactic defibrillator implantation in patients with nonischemic dilated cardiomyopathy. N Engl J Med 2004;350:2151–8.

[37] Rashba EJ, Lamas GA, Couderc JP, Hollist SM, Dzavik V, Ruzyllo W, et al. Electrophysiological effects of late percutaneous coronary intervention for infarct-related coronary artery occlusion: the Occluded Artery Trial-Electrophysiological Mechanisms (OAT-EP). Circulation 2009;119:779–87.

[38] Moss AJ. MADIT-I and MADIT-II. J Cardiovasc Electrophysiol 2003;14:S96–8.

[39] Moss AJ, Brown MW, Cannom DS, Daubert JP, Estes M, Foster E, et al. Multicenter automatic defibrillator implantation trial-cardiac resynchronization therapy (MADIT-CRT): design and clin-ical protocol. Ann Noninvasive Electrocardiol 2005;10:34–43.

[40] Couderc JP, Garnett C, Li M, Handzel R, McNitt S, Xia X, et al. Highly Automated QT Measurement Techniques in 7 Thorough QT Studies Implemented under ICH E14 Guidelines. Ann Noninvasive Electrocardiol 2011;16:13–24.

[41] Darpo B, Fossa AA, Couderc JP, Zhou M, Schreyer A, Ticktin M, et al. Improving the precision of QT measurements. Cardiol J 2011;18:401–10.

[42] Khawaja A, Petrovic R, Safer A, Baas T, Dossel O, Fischer R. Analyzing Thorough QT Study 1 & 2 in the Telemetric and Holter ECG Warehouse (THEW) using Hannover ECG System HES: A validation study. Comput Cardiol (2010) 2010;37:349–52.

[43] Xiao Jie, Rodriguez B, Pueyo E. A new ECG biomarker for drug toxicity: a combined signal pro-cessing and computational modeling study, Engineering in Medicine and Biology Society (EMBS), 2010 Annual International Conference of the IEEE, Vol, pp. 2565–68.

[44] Abrahamsson C, Dota C, Skallefell B, Carlsson L, Halawani D, Frison L, et al. DeltaT50–a new method to assess temporal ventricular repolarization variability. J Electrocardiol 2011;44:477–9.

[45] Burattini L, Zareba W, Burattini R. Identification of gender-related normality regions for T-wave alternans. Ann Noninvasive Electrocardiol 2010;15:328–36.

[46] Couderc JP, Xia X, Peterson DR, McNitt S, Zhao H, Polonsky S, et al. T-wave morphology abnor-malities in benign, potent, and arrhythmogenic I(kr) inhibition. Heart Rhythm 2011;8:1036–43.

[47] Sassi R, Mainardi LT. An estimate of the dispersion of repolarization times based on a biophysical model of the ECG. IEEE Trans Biomed Eng 2011;58:3396–405.

Path to Regulatory Qualification Process Development

18

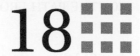

Path to Regulatory Qualification Program Development: A US FDA Perspective

Shashi Amur

OFFICE OF TRANSLATIONAL SCIENCES, CENTER FOR DRUG EVALUATION AND RESEARCH, FOOD AND DRUG ADMINISTRATION, SILVER SPRING, MARYLAND, USA

The US Food and Drug Administration (FDA) has long recognized the importance of the development and use of biomarkers in improving the drug development process [1–3]. In order to encourage the use of exploratory biomarkers in this process, a voluntary genomic data submission (VGDS) process was set up in 2004, which was expanded to voluntary exploratory data submission (VXDS) in 2006. This process led to the submission of over 50 VXDSs in a number of therapeutic areas, and allowed scientific exchange between the VXDS submitters and the FDA. Some of these VXDS submissions were evaluated jointly by the FDA and European Medicines Agency (EMA). The experience gained from this process has helped FDA in understanding the strategies and tools used by the sponsors in the generation and analysis of biomarker data and also in developing new policy. The VXDS process has provided an opportunity for the sponsors to better understand FDA's perspective on biomarker data and analyses as well as the application of lessons learned from the VXDS process to drug development [4,5].

The use of biomarkers in drug development has increased over the years in multiple ways: as exploratory biomarkers (e.g., to understand the mechanism of action of the drug); in clinical trial design (e.g., stratification, dose selection and patient selection); and in drug and biomarker co-development. However, broad acceptance of a biomarker in the regulatory process of drug development and approval (Investigational New Drug/New Drug Application/Biologics License Application (IND/NDA/BLA)) occurs over a long time frame and in the context of a single drug. While this remains a valuable pathway, there is a need for a more efficient pathway to qualify biomarkers for use in the development of multiple drugs. The identification of the need to provide a framework for the development and regulatory acceptance of scientific tools for use in drug development programs led to the establishment of a pilot project for biomarker qualification.

The first submission for biomarker qualification was from the Predictive Safety Testing Consortium (PSTC), and this was initiated through the VXDS process as a joint submission to FDA and EMA for the qualification of seven urinary biomarkers as predictors of drug-mediated nephrotoxicity [6]. The review team at FDA and EMA evaluated the data and identified data gaps in the initial submission leading to additional work by the consortium and evaluation by the review teams. In 2008, the urinary kidney biomarkers (KIM-1, Albumin, Total Protein, β2-Microglobulin, Cystatin C, Clusterin and Trefoil factor-3) were qualified for the detection of acute drug-induced nephrotoxicity in rats in conjunction with traditional clinical chemistry markers and histology in toxicology studies.

The experience gained with the pilot process led to a careful evaluation of the steps involved in the process, and subsequent introduction of the Biomarker Qualification Program in 2009. This effort is one component of the Drug Development Tool (DDT) Qualification Program established by Center for Drug Evaluation and Research (CDER) as an outgrowth of the FDA's Critical Path Initiative. A draft guidance entitled, 'Qualification Process for Drug Development Tools' was issued in 2010 [7] and a public website on 'Drug Development Tools' was made available in late 2011 [8] that defines qualification and provides a list of qualification programs available at CDER, FDA.

CDER's Biomarker Qualification Program has dedicated personnel to manage and streamline the program: Program co-Directors, a Science Coordinator and a Regulatory Project Manager. The goals of the Biomarker Qualification Program are to:

1) Provide a framework for scientific development and regulatory acceptance of biomarkers for use in drug development.
2) Facilitate integration of qualified biomarkers in the regulatory review process.
3) Encourage the identification of new and emerging biomarkers for evaluation and utilization in regulatory decision-making.
4) Support outreach to relevant external stakeholders to foster biomarker development.

The Biomarker Qualification Process at US FDA

The biomarker qualification process at FDA can be divided into an Initiation stage, Consultation and Advice stage, and Review stage (Fig. 18.1).

Initiation stage: The submitter's scientific and administrative readiness for proceeding to enter into the biomarker qualification (BQ) process, is assessed in the initiation stage and advice provided, if needed. After the receipt of the Letter of Intent (LOI) from the submitter containing information on the biomarkers to be qualified including the proposed context of use of the biomarkers, CDER assesses the LOI and determines whether to proceed to the next step of biomarker qualification, i.e., formation of interdisciplinary biomarker qualification review team (BQRT).
Consultation and Advice stage: The consultation and advice stage begins with the formation of a BQRT. The LOI is reviewed by the BQRT and comments/advice provided by the BQRT is sent to the submitters. The next step is the submission of the Initial Briefing Package by the submitters that describes the biomarker(s) proposed for qualification, full context of biomarker use, rationale for its use in drug development; provides preliminary data relevant to the biomarker(s) as well as an

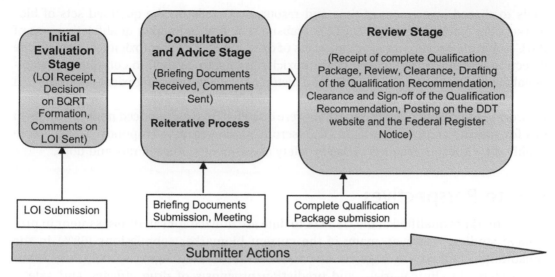

FIGURE 18.1 Biomarker Qualification process at US FDA

analysis of the knowledge gaps; and describes the development plan for the biomarker. This package is reviewed by the BQRT and comments sent to the submitter as 'Preliminary Advice' prior to meeting with the submitter. Major issues identified by the submitter and BQRT are discussed in addition to next steps needed. This is an iterative process, which continues until the knowledge gaps are addressed and all necessary evidence to support the qualification of biomarkers for the specified context of use is ready to be submitted to BQRT.

Review Stage: The review stage begins with the receipt of the full qualification package, and includes a detailed review of the evidence provided, written discipline-specific reviews and clearance from the respective offices/divisions and the Biomarker Qualification Program directors. This stage ends with the authoring of a Draft Qualification Recommendation (QR) by the BQRT. The Draft QR is cleared by relevant management officials at CDER and is signed off by the Center Director. A Federal Register Notice about the Draft QR will be posted to enable receipt of public comments. After the comment period has ended, a final QR will be issued. This final QR is posted as an appendix to the DDT Qualification Process guidance.

Current Status of Biomarker Qualification Submissions

Currently, fourteen biomarker qualification submissions are in the consultation and advice stage, one submission is in the review stage, and three sets of biomarkers have been qualified. Based on the current submissions, consortia appear to be the most efficient path for biomarker development; possibly due to the collaborative format, which leads to shared investment of time and resources. Details on the qualified sets of bio-markers are available on the FDA DDT website. The first biomarker qualification was of PSTC-submitted seven urinary biomarkers of drug-induced nephrotoxicity in 2008 for the detection of acute drug-induced nephrotoxicity in rats, to be used to complement traditional clinical chemistry marker data and histopathology findings in toxicology studies. In 2010, urinary Clusterin and Renal Papillary Antigen (RPA-1) submitted by Health and Environmental Sciences Institute (HESI) were qualified for drug-induced nephrotoxicity in rats for specific contexts of use. In 2012, serum/plasma cardiac Troponins T and I were qualified for specific contexts of use in safety assessment studies in rats and dogs.

Future Perspectives

The biomarkers qualified at the US FDA to date are utilized for safety assessment in pre-clinical studies. However, many of the current biomarker submissions (68%) in the consultation and advice stage are associated with disease diagnosis, inclusion/exclusion criteria in clinical trials, and prediction/prognosis of drug efficacy and safety. Thus, biomarkers qualified in the coming years may be used in different stages of clinical trials (Phases 1, 2 and 3). Consortia are likely to remain a favorable pathway to move exploratory biomarkers to application in drug development, because of the investment of resources and collaborative leveraging needed for this effort. Key factors leading to successful outcomes include early communication with the FDA Biomarker Qualification Program group, well-defined biomarker(s) and a clear description of the context of use in drug development. Qualified biomarkers are likely to facilitate the development of new therapeutics in multiple ways: by predicting toxicity or long term outcomes; by identifying patients likely to respond; by identifying patients at risk of developing adverse reactions; and also by reducing the time and cost of the drug development process.

■ ■ Disclaimer ■

The views expressed in this chapter are those of the authors and do not necessarily reflect the official views of FDA.

Acknowledgments

The author would like to thank ShaAvhree Buckman-Garner, MD., Ph.D., F.A.A.P., Marc Walton, MD. Ph.D., and Marianne Noone, R.N., for their critical review of the manuscript and helpful suggestions.

References

[1] http://www.fda.gov/downloads/ScienceResearch/SpecialTopics/CriticalPathInitiative/CriticalPath OpportunitiesReports/ucm113411.pdf. Date accessed June 7, 2013.

[2] FDA Critical Path Opportunities List. http://www.fda.gov/downloads/ScienceResearch/Special Topics/CriticalPathInitiative/CriticalPathOpportunitiesReports/UCM077258.pdf; 2006. Accessed June 7, 2013.

[3] Amur S, Frueh FW, Lesko LJ, Huang S-M. Integration and use of biomarkers in drug development, regulation and clinical practice: a US regulatory perspective. Biomarkers Med 2008;2(3):305–11.

[4] Goodsaid FM, Amur S, Aubrecht J, Burczynski ME, Carl K, Catalano J, et al. Voluntary exploratory data submissions to the US FDA and the EMA: experience and impact. Nat Rev Drug Discov 2010; 9(6):435–45.

[5] Woodcock J, Buckman S, Goodsaid F, Walton MK, Zineh I. Qualifying biomarkers for use in drug development: a US Food and Drug Administration overview. Expert Opin Med Diagn 2011;5(5): 369–73.

[6] Goodsaid, F., and Papaluca, M. Evolution of biomarker qualification at the health authorities. Nat Biotechnol 28(5): 441–443.

[7] FDA Guidance for Industry: Qualification Process for Drug Development Tools http://www.fda.gov/downloads/Drugs/GuidanceComplianceRegulatoryInformation/Guidances/UCM230597.pdf

[8] FDA Biomarker Qualification Program- Website http://www.fda.gov/Drugs/DevelopmentApproval Process/DrugDevelopmentToolsQualificationProgram/ucm284076.htm

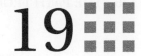
Path to Regulatory Qualification Process Development

Yasuto Otsubo, Akihiro Ishiguro, Yoshiaki Uyama

PMDA OMICS PROJECT (POP), PHARMACEUTICALS AND MEDICAL DEVICES AGENCY (PMDA), JAPAN

The PMDA Omics Project (POP; formerly known as the Pharmacogenomics Discussion Group (PDG), see Chapter 4 for more information) has been actively working to promote pharmacogenomics (PGx)- and biomarker-based drug and device development. POP has also had many informal meetings with industry and/or academia to understand the latest scientific information relating to 'omics'. In 2007, POP joined the US Food and Drug Administration (US-FDA) and the European Medicine Agency (EMA) Joint Voluntary Exploratory Data Submission meetings (J-VXDS), as an observer. However, in the above activities, there was no formal process for providing PMDA's comments and reports to industry or academia. Thus, the need to strengthen PMDA's contribution in PGx- and biomarker-based drug and device developments, taking into consideration regulatory harmonization was recognized. In April 2009, PMDA created a formal process of scientific consultation focusing on PGx/biomarker qualification. There are two main purposes for this consultation. One is to discuss appropriate drug and device development strategies using PGx/biomarkers for regulatory submissions. The other is to evaluate biomarker data for regulatory qualification. This process will also promote collaborative biomarker qualification between PMDA and other regulatory agencies such as US-FDA and EMA [1,2], since these agencies have similar processes for biomarker qualification. Through this consultation, PMDA aims to maximize the efficiency of drug/device development and to promote the use of personalized medicine in clinical practice.

Fig. 19.1 shows the standard timeline for biomarker qualification, which is generally completed within 24 weeks. However, this timeline is flexible, and may vary according to the situation or outcome of the consultation. At the end of the consultation, an official assessment report is provided by PMDA.

In FY2009, the Predictive Safety Testing Consortium (PSTC) submitted data for seven urinary biomarkers for nephrotoxicity (cystatin C, β2-microglobulin, total protein, clusterin, KIM-1, TFF3, and albumin) to PMDA in order to seek PMDA's agreement with the contexts of the proposed biomarkers and to discuss the future qualification strategies for the biomarkers. The official assessment report from PMDA for this consultation is available on the PMDA website [3] and the conclusions are summarized in Table 19.1.

The final conclusion of PMDA is similar to the conclusions reported by US-FDA and EMA [4,5]. Therefore, these seven biomarkers, for use within the specific context, 'to

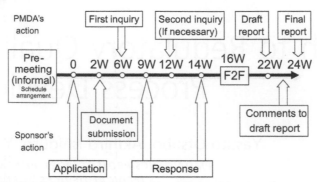

FIGURE 19.1 Standard timeline for the consultation on biomarker qualification. The pre-meeting is usually held to confirm the consultation schedule. After the application, first and second, if necessary, inquiries will be sent from PMDA. The consultation is generally completed within 24 weeks.

detect drug-induced acute urinary tubular changes or acute glomerular changes/injury in rat Good Laboratory Practice (GLP) studies', are now qualified at the same level by the core regulatory agencies in the International Conference on Harmonization of Technical Requirements for Registration of Pharmaceuticals for Human Use (ICH). International qualification will facilitate the use of biomarkers in drug and device developments, particularly in the current era of globalization and will also promote the global accumulation of scientific evidence, contributing to better regulatory assessments and decisions. Therefore, biomarker qualifications should be conducted at the international level, and not by one regulatory agency alone. For that purpose, the ICH E16 guideline entitled 'Biomarkers related to drug or biotechnology product development: context, structure and format of qualification submissions' implemented in January 2011 in Japan [6] will facilitate simultaneous global data submission for biomarker qualifications.

To increase the efficiency of drug/device development, and to achieve the goals of personalized medicine in clinical practice, more biomarkers need to be internationally qualified. The role of scientific consortia is very important in rapidly accumulating scientific data for biomarker qualification, as significant resources are needed to accomplish

Table 19.1 Summary of the PMDA Conclusions

- It is important to confirm the qualification of novel biomarkers (BMs) for their objective and context of use, prior to widely using novel BMs in drug developments.
- The PSTC data regarding seven BMs (Kim-1, clusterin, albumin, TFF3, cystatin C, β2-microglobulin and total protein) will be useful for new drug developments.
- The use of these 7 BMs is acceptable for the purpose of detecting drug-induced acute urinary tubular changes or acute glomerular changes/injury in rat GLP studies when they are used in combination with existing BMs (serum creatinine and blood urea nitrogen (BUN)).
- Sufficient qualification has not been performed for general wide use of these seven novel BMs for the detection of drug-induced acute kidney injury in early clinical studies (Phase I studies, etc.). The utility of these BMs should be individually judged on the basis of results obtained in the courses of future clinical developments of drugs or future biomarker qualifications.

this, and because these resources may be beyond the reach of a single company or an academic laboratory. In Japan, the Japan PGx Data Science Consortium (JPDSC) [7] was established in February 2009 to identify a genetic association factor with serious adverse events. Within the consortium, Japanese pharmaceutical companies have worked together to establish a control DNA database for the Japanese population. On the regulatory side, PMDA has worked to strengthen and build collaborative relations with US-FDA and EMA to further promote international harmonization on PGx and biomarker qualification. In 2012, PMDA started a new category of scientific consultation on PGx/biomarker qualification to provide more opportunities for industry and academia [8]. In this new category, PMDA encourages experts from industry and academia to visit the PMDA more frequently not only for data qualification, but also for planning the design of biomarker qualification studies, and for following up on past consultation items.

It is expected that these efforts will help to make personalized medicine a reality in daily practice.

Acknowledgment

The views expressed in this chapter are those of the authors and do not necessarily reflect the official views of Pharmaceuticals and Medical Devices Agency.

References

[1] US-Food and Drug Administration, Biomarker qualification process, http://www.fda.gov/Drugs/DevelopmentApprovalProcess/DrugDevelopmentToolsQualificationProgram/ucm284076.htm (Accessed on June 14, 2013)

[2] European Medicine Agency, Qualification of novel methodology for medicine development. http://www.ema.europa.eu/ema/index.jsp?curl=pages/regulation/document_listing/document_listing_000319.jsp&mid=WC0b01ac0580022bb0 (Accessed on June 14, 2013).

[3] Pharmaceuticals and Medical Devices Agency, Record of the Consultation on Pharmacogenomics/Biomarkers, http://www.pmda.go.jp/operations/shonin/info/consult/file/pbm-kiroku-e.pdf (Accessed on June 14, 2013).

[4] US-Food and Drug Administration, Review submission of the qualification of seven biomarkers of drug-induced nephrotoxicity in rats. http://www.fda.gov/downloads/Drugs/DevelopmentApprovalProcess/DrugDevelopmentToolsQualificationProgram/UCM285031.pdf (Accessed on June 14, 2013).

[5] European Medicine Agency, Final conclusions on the pilot joint emea/fda vxds experience on qualification of nephrotoxicity biomarkers. http://www.ema.europa.eu/docs/en_GB/document_library/Regulatory_and_procedural_guideline/2009/10/WC500004205.pdf (Accessed on June 14, 2013).

[6] Ministry of Health, Labour and Welfare, ICH-E16 guideline; Biomarkers Related to Drug or Biotechnology Product Development: Context, Structure and Format of Qualification Submissions, Notification No. 0120–1/0120–1, 2011. http://www.pmda.go.jp/ich/e/e16_11_1_20.pdf (Accessed on June 14, 2013).

[7] Japan PGx data science consortium, http://www.jpdsc.org/ (Accessed on June 14, 2013).

[8] Pharmaceuticals and Medical Devices Agency, Process of scientific consultation on pharmacogenomics/biomarker. http://www.pmda.go.jp/operations/shonin/info/consult/file/0302070-betten4.pdf (Accessed on June 14, 2013).

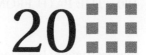

20

The Tortuous Path From Development to Qualification of Biomarkers

Federico Goodsaid

STRATEGIC REGULATORY INTELLIGENCE, REGULATORY AFFAIRS, VERTEX PHARMACEUTICALS, WASHINGTON, DC, USA

The chapters in this book share a link to two parallel experiences in the search for better tools for the development of new and better therapies. One is an outcome of the work summarized in these chapters: the current processes that lead from biomarker development to qualification for regulatory use. The other one is the path by which regulatory agencies in the US, Europe and Japan developed these processes, at once imperfect, but also essential. Both experiences have been complex and difficult.

The decade over which these processes were developed was also a decade in which regulatory agencies identified the need for a collaborative and proactive approach to interacting with pharmaceutical companies. The transformation over the past decade has been not so much about how drugs are studied or how drug submissions are reviewed, but about whether successful drug development and accurate regulatory review may continue to be viewed as independent, and often mutually adversarial, activities. A reduction in this adversarial relationship is reflected in several areas, but the single most important area for collaborative discussions between companies and agencies has been the interpretation of biomarker measurements. Regulatory agencies in the US, Europe, and Japan (FDA, EMA, and PMDA) have, over the past decade, encouraged discussions about exploratory biomarker data in Voluntary Exploratory Data Submissions (VXDS) which predated the development of biomarker qualification processes. Biomarker qualification processes are both the beginning of new regulatory processes and also the continuation of initiatives started several years before these processes were proposed.

In the end, it is the renewed focus on the science itself that is really transformative for interactions with regulatory agencies. A focus on science has an impact not only on specific regulatory decisions, but also on the experience of developing a new therapy and sharing the clinical data for this novel therapy with regulatory agencies. Biomarkers are an integral part of the lexicon for these discussions. Their regulatory qualification is needed to expand the value of these discussions. It is exciting to see how even the initial modest boundaries for the context of use in the nonclinical qualification of biomarkers of nephrotoxicity have led to discussions in regulatory submissions about their value for an accurate assessment of risk.

As we move beyond some of these early successes with biomarker qualification processes, we can also sense some major challenges. Even in the absence of regulatory guidance, it seems reflexive for regulatory reviewers to expect minimum levels for contexts of use to be met by a set of evidentiary standards, rather than for minimum levels of evidentiary standards to be met by a set of contexts of use. The gap between these two approaches is the difference between a dynamic incremental process for biomarker qualification as opposed to a static biomarker qualification process not likely to succeed. The experience gained thus far in these regulatory processes should emphasize the match of a regulatory context of use for qualification to the available data and to guide the drafting of documents with which those interested in qualifying biomarkers can accurately assess the boundaries for the context of use of their submissions.

In addition to summarizing experience in the pharmaceutical industry in biomarker development and qualification, the chapters in this book also summarize two major biomarker research areas: toxicogenomics and drug safety. These two areas were chosen because they populated much of the early biomarker qualification submissions to the FDA, EMA and PMDA, and because they explicitly show the long-term impact that biomarker qualification is expected to have on biomarker research: biomarkers which can be qualified through a straightforward regulatory process are also likely to be more intensively sought after in pharmaceutical research and development.

Other chapters in this book summarize the challenges of consortia which have carried most of the burden in the submission of data for biomarker qualification. The difficult work of consortia is considered from afar as an excellent example of collaboration between the pharmaceutical industry and academic and regulatory scientists. However, as the chapters in this section show, these collaborations are effective only if consortium members are actively engaged in the goals of these consortia. This active engagement is not always achieved, and is closely related to the incremental success shown by consortia. In the specific example of biomarker qualification, an incremental regulatory qualification process is important for the long-term success of consortium collaboration.

The future for the development and qualification of biomarkers will be bright, not necessarily because there will ever be enough funds to support them, but because better therapies will not reach the market without them. Budgets for biomarkers in industry and government may not cover funding needs for these in the immediate future. What we can be sure about today is that, while we may not know what a definitive universal process for regulatory biomarker qualification will look like, there will be one.

Index

Note: Page numbers followed by "f" denote figures; "t" tables; and "b" boxes.

Printed and bound by CPI Group (UK) Ltd, Croydon, CR0 4YY

03/10/2024

01040315-0009